THE LIFE CHANGING POWER OF LATIN DANCE

How Latin Dance Builds the Ultimate Woman: Strength Through Feminity, Confidence, Passion and Happiness

BY LIZ LIRA

Dance Forever! ~ Liz Lira

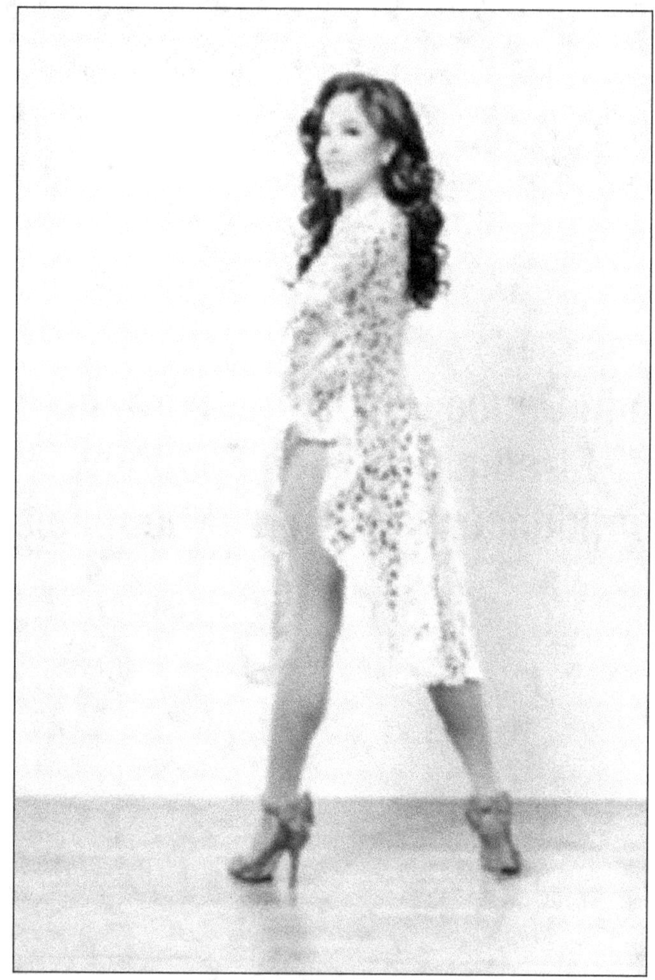

Live the life you always desired and believe in yourself!
Liz Lira

V. 2 Copyright 2023
Liz Lira Enterprises, Inc
All Rights Reserved
ISBN: 979-8878367-16-5

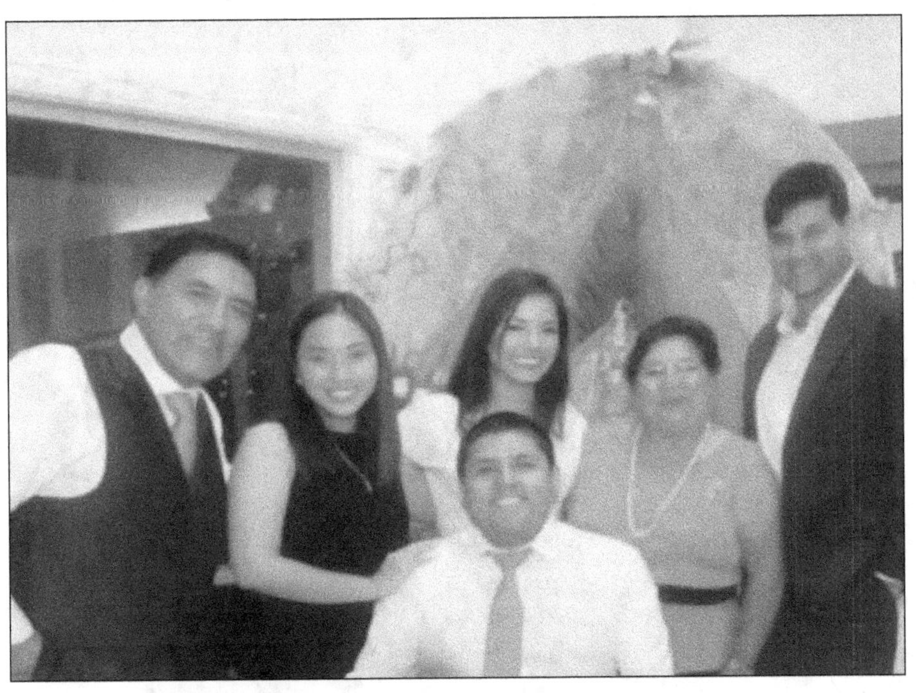

My beautiful loving family. From Left to Right …
Juan, Paulina, Kevin, Liz, Celina, and Reef

My gorgeous son. Dream Lira Karim

DEDICATION

To my incredible family, my Rock and Strength, Celina, Kevin, Juan, Pauline, and my grandmother Alicia – You are my heart.

And my best friend Reef- You inspire me to be the woman I have always wanted to be. You are my Soul. I love you so much. You are my World.

Beth Burns, founder of Saint Joseph Ballet Company. Thank you for saving my life.

Dear Friends: Steve Alas, Marina Valencia, Gary Forman and Kerim Soyoguz- Thank you for bringing me back to life.

To my amazing students and friends - Thank you for believing in me and giving me the honor to share dance with you.

DISCLAIMER

I want to share with you my incredible journey, as an immigrant, and a glimpse of my dance experience and how those experiences have shaped who I am today. I am excited to share with you how dance has impacted my life by showing me the world, meeting the most incredible people from all levels of society, everlasting fairytale memories and most importantly, how dance absolutely changed my personal life and relationships.

All thoughts, exercises, comments in this book are my ideas based on my dance experience and personal training. As I am not a doctor, please consult your physician for any medical questions on health and fitness.

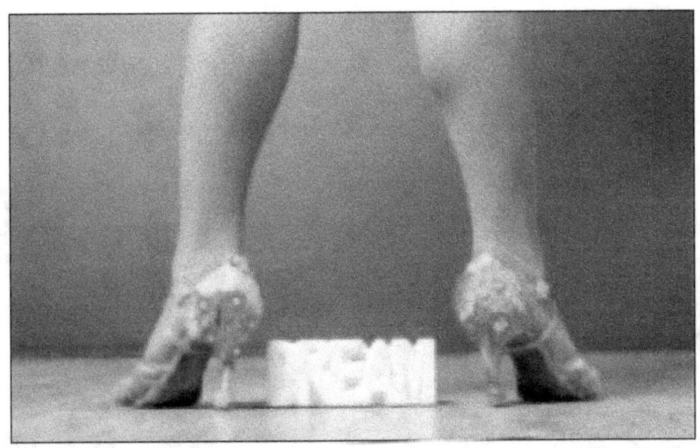

Dreams Come True! ~ Liz Lira

TABLE OF CONTENTS

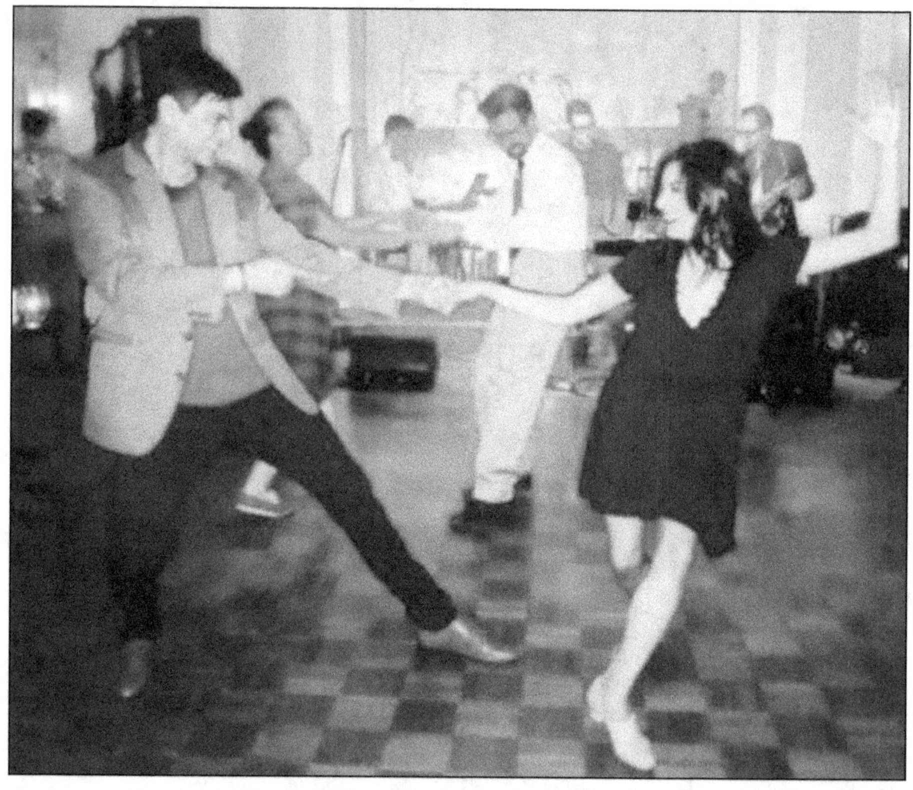

The Connection of Dance
Liz Lira and Reef Karim Swing dancing the night away at Clifton's
in Los Angeles, Ca

xi

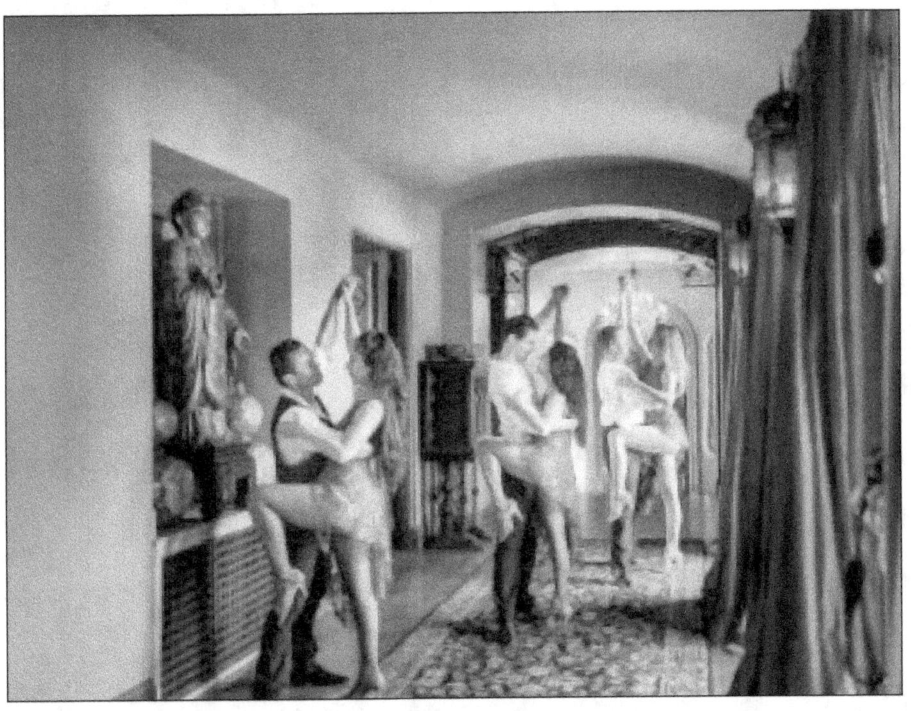

Liz Lira Dance Academy featured dancers at Travel Magazine-
Taste of the World!
Dancers Jose Mendosei, Natalia Romo, Michael Zazarino, Liz Lira,
Brian Lee, and Lexi Quintero.
Photo credit @Rareperspective

**Free Salsa and Bachata
Online Videos**

This book includes videos and interviews with
dance tips, instruction, and guidance.

Go here: www.lizlira.com

PROLOGUE BY SHIRLEY BALLAS

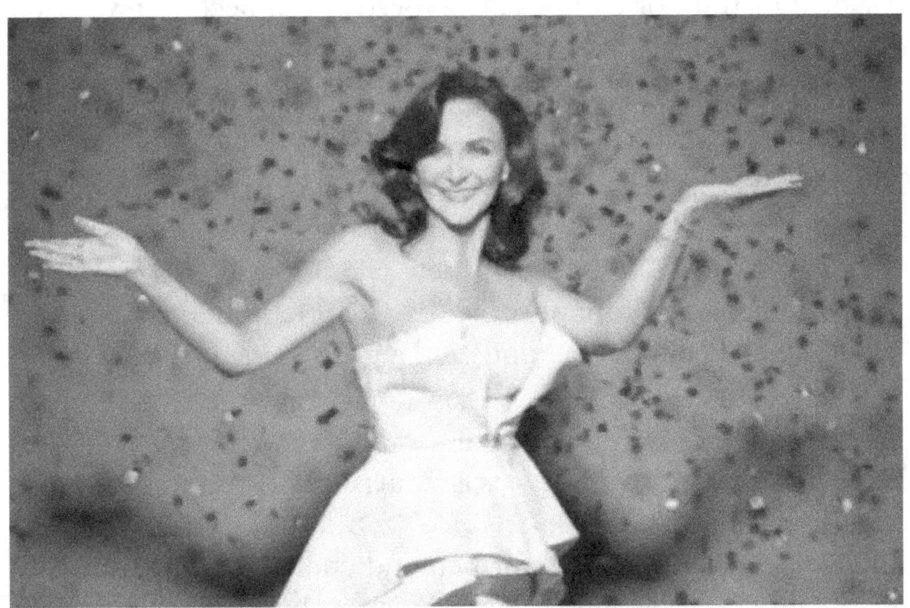

Former World Latin Champion Shirley Ballas
Judge: The British Dance Show: Strictly Come Dancing

I remember the first time I met Liz Lira in 2007. I have seen everything in professional dance. As a world champion Latin dancer, myself, and a champion ballroom dance coach, I have seen it all. But there was something different about Liz; her grace, her poise, her positivity, her immense work ethic; the combination was fascinating to me.

I worked with Liz for a few years and saw her quickly grow in all aspects of dance, dance techniques, specific technical elements, footwork, performance, styling and all the minute details that differentiate a world champion from other dancers who are simply left wanting.

Liz has such a sturdy foundation of positivity, musicality, and love for dance. It took me a while to realize she did not just love to perform or train or compete, she loved to connect, to grow as a person from dance.

I could not think of a better person to write this book than Liz Lira. She's a world champion dancer, a champion dance coach, and a champion personal coach; all wrapped in a petite package of powerful women who can spin like a top.

And she's really onto something.

The idea that a strong woman is also a feminine woman is a lesson we all need to remember and a timely lesson at that.

I've believed in Liz since I first met her, and her achievements match her drive and talent; she's worked as a choreographer on *Dancing with the Stars*. She was a recurring choreographer on the television show *So You Think You Can Dance* and Liz performed on *Star Search* and has performed and choreographed on many feature films, television shows and big stage performances around the world.

I'm so proud of her for taking her dance experience, life experience, and personal coaching experience to write this especially important book.

Keep Dancing!!

Shirley Ballas

Judge: Strictly Come Dancing

World Latin Champion

British Ballroom Champion

CHAPTER 1

WHO AM I AND WHY SHOULD YOU LISTEN TO ME?

Hi, I'm Liz Lira.

I'm a world champion Latin dancer, a strong feminine woman, and a personal lifestyle coach empowering women to build strength and confidence through femininity, and empowering med to become stronger leaders in life, all through the art of Latin dance and movement.

I have dedicated my life to spreading the power of dance to not just build better dancers, but to build better people. Dance heals. Dance builds confidence. Dance builds trust. Dance builds connection. Dance builds body awareness and acceptance.

Partner dancing is an incredibly powerful personal development experience that many people haven't discovered yet.

And my wish for you, as you read this book, is to add partner dancing to your life.

The world is changing quickly. People are focusing more on social issues. Women are growing stronger by the second.

And both men and women are navigating the tricky waters of relationships, roles, communication, and trust.

Divorce is higher than ever. Many successful women are alone. Many successful men are lonely.

And I get asked questions like these all the time:

What is a strong woman?

Is chivalry dead?

Why can't men be more like women?

Why can't women be more like men?

Well, the reality is that men and women are different; and that's a great thing.

Both sexes can be strong in their own way.

I believe that a strong woman is equal but also feminine. Women are not men; they should never be men; equality does not mean being like a man; it means being a strong woman, making your own choices and expressing your femininity.

Woman should be women. Men should be men. But we can learn to trust each other, communicate with each other, connect with each other *on the dance floor* in a safe place to strengthen our ability *off the dance floor.*

I've learned to become a strong, feminine, successful woman and I owe much of my success to the skills I learned in the art and experience of Latin dance.

I've had the opportunity to experience all types of dances at an exceedingly high level, training with the top teachers in the world in Ballet, Jazz, Flamenco, Latin, Ballroom, Argentine Tango, and Salsa.

And I've been able to pioneer and innovate a new style of Salsa (adding ballroom, ballet, and partnering technique focusing on weight distribution and body awareness to create better lines, better turns, better tricks, and more fun social dancing).

But, just as important, if not more, I've developed a method (The Liz Lira Method) to train people to become better dancers but also to become better people by building confidence, trust, intimacy, body awareness, styling, and connection.

I could help couples build more intimacy and connection.

I help men become stronger leaders, more confident and more desirable to women.

And I can help women bask in their femininity while building trust, connection, body awareness and confidence in themselves and their abilities.

Now before I share my story, I want to thank you for reading my book and investing some of your precious time to learn about the power of Latin Dance.

You won't regret it. It's a life changer.

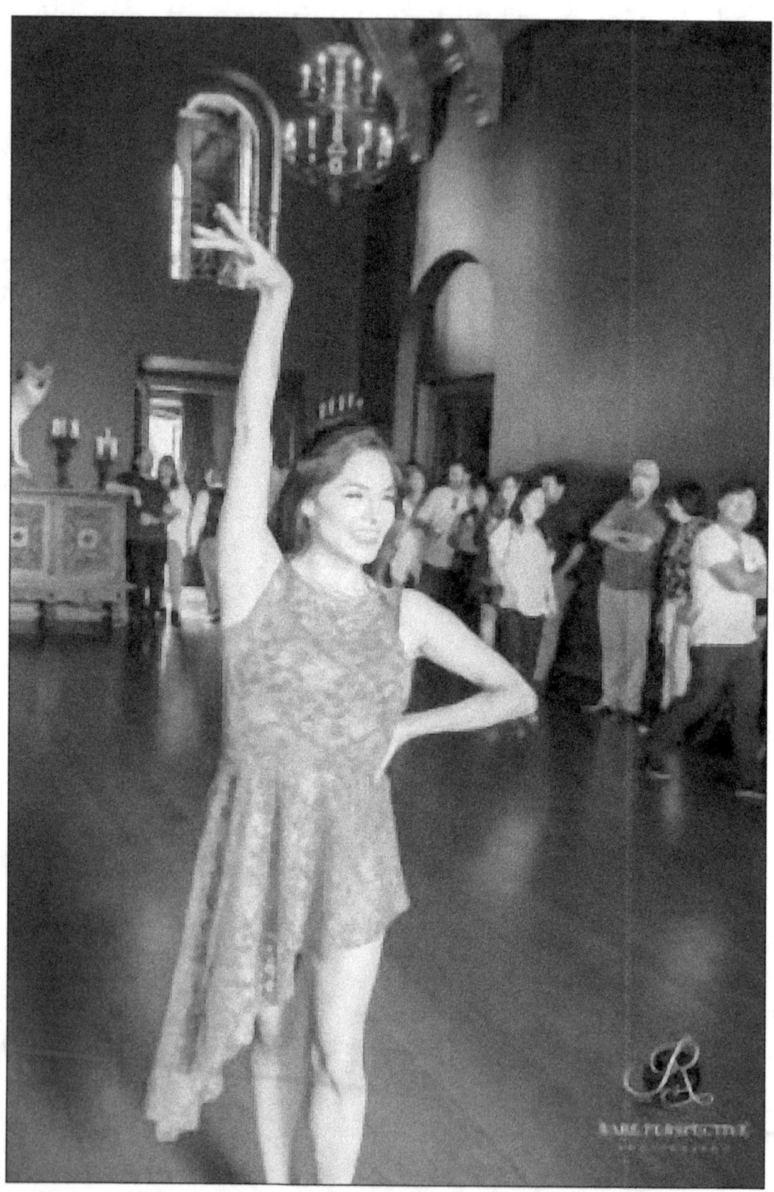

Liz Lira Travel Magazine featured artist at Paramount Estate in Los Angeles, Ca One of my favorite venues in LA.
Photo credit: @Rareperspective

CHAPTER 2

I COULD HAVE BEEN ANOTHER STATISTIC

"Run! Find the fire so you can breathe."

At the age of six, my eyes are red, and I can't stop crying. I couldn't breathe. It was tear gas that had been thrown into our home by the rebels. I remember my mom holding my hand while we ran as fast as we could upstairs to the rooftop of our building. Our neighbors had created a bonfire so we could sit around it to keep warm.

That was my last memory of my difficult and challenging life in my home country, La Paz, Bolivia.

I was born a premature baby at seven months. I barely made it into this world. My eyes and mouth were shut. My dad says I was the size of his palm. My dear grandfather Juan had to use his house as collateral for my medical bill payments so the hospital could keep me alive in the incubator. What a miraculous way to enter this world.

I grew up in a very disciplined home focused on strong education from a noticeably early age. I remember doing a year's worth of school material during my summer break at the age of six. I was very shy, was taught not to talk back, do as I'm told, and always show good behavior.

And I want to be completely transparent, I suffered immensely and had an exceedingly difficult childhood. I had become so depressed; I had cut my left wrist hoping to die at the age of six. I still have the scar to this day.

I saw women abused as they were forced to stay home, take care of their children, cook, clean, and wait for their husbands to return, without ever thinking for themselves. That could have been me! Even so, this was my path and I now love the place of my birth and have never forgotten my roots. Family first, all for one and one for all.

I had discipline in my upbringing with a focus on school and was told that hard work pays off. Respect yourself and those around you. Profound principles for a six-year-old.

My mom, Celina, was a young mom. She helped her mom raise all five brothers and sisters. One of the hardest working and dedicated women I've ever met. She ran a couple of restaurants and toy stores while taking care of me. Wow! From an early age, I was introduced to multi-tasking, being organized, keeping things clean, not being lazy (she would always have something for me to do after I was done with my homework) and always doing the right thing. I always look up to her and think of her when I start feeling lazy.

Fearless child. Yes, that's me! I used to jump off buildings, windows, bikes, anything really. I remember sliding down a four-story building stair railing and falling onto hard cement face down; my upper forehead landed on a bow rake. I still have that scar too. We rode the bus often and when I was bored, I would open the doors and hang off the side of the bus to feel the air on my face. You name it, I've either done it or wanted to do it. I've always had a sense of adventure, curiosity, and exploring of all things.

Every day, all around me, since the day I was born, I grew up listening to the most beautiful music called Tropical music (Salsa, Merengue, Cumbia, Cha-cha-cha, Danzon,) Boleros, and Argentine Tango. I was amazed that at family parties, my family would always have a live Salsa and Tango/Ballads orchestra. Music was always a part of me. The children were always encouraged to dance and learn routines using pop culture dance moves that were popular that year. Like the Macarena or Bolivian traditional dances.

Although Bolivia is a third world country and life is rough with a lot of poverty and corruption, many people live a happy life and celebrate each other. It's all about family. We had all kinds of family gatherings with lots of food and amazing music. I would dance every day at school, at home before going to bed and at weekend parties. It definitely made life a little more joyful.

My uncles in their youth had created a Disco/ R&B dance group called Grupo X (group X) and my mom took me to watch them in the finals. They were fast, sharp, athletic, and well-coordinated. Simply delightful and super clean. They won!! The family was so proud. My uncles were good men. Because they had dance in their life, they were able to build their self-esteem and confidence. Yet stay humble and be good men as well.

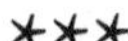

It was destiny or a fortuitous event in my life, but I always carried the heavy weight on my shoulders of my mom and dad leaving everything behind in the pursuit of a better life for me "The American Dream." I've done everything in my power to give back to my family and ensure they have a happy life in our home in America.

Just before our departure, my mom was seven months pregnant, and a car hit the bus we were in, and the baby had the umbilical cord wrapped around itself and died. So tragic. My mom could have died too. She had no idea the baby died in her stomach. She was so sick, but thankfully she went to the hospital in time to get the baby out and get her back to normal. I thank God everyday my mommy was saved, and I never forgot our little angel in heaven.

Coming to America gave us inspiration, hope for a better life and the promise of a land of opportunity. I remember flying in an airplane and crossing the border in a car. We stayed with family and eventually moved into someone's guest house. It was incredibly challenging to adapt to a new culture, language, and laws. Laws? Coming from a corrupt country where anything goes, we weren't used to laws. We had to face a new world, America. In Bolivia, people did whatever they want, pay off police officers to get away with things, high rate of women getting abused, and no one says anything.

The hardest part was the language barrier. In elementary school, I had the hardest time meshing with the other children in school because I didn't know how to stand up for myself. So, I became a muted child, and as a result, I became more introverted. We couldn't afford fashionable clothes or brand labels, so I would go to school with simple clothes that didn't really fit me.

School was super hard. I was bullied as a young child. Learning a new language, I struggled to communicate clearly. It was easy to pick on me because I didn't defend myself. I didn't know how, and I didn't want to get in trouble. I remember crying every day. The only thing I knew best was to study and do my homework. I have never forgotten how it felt to be put down, picked on and treated like an animal.

✶✶✶

"5-6-7-8. Demi-pile, arms in first position and chin up."

At the age of six and a half, I auditioned for a non-profit organization called Saint Joseph Ballet Company, founded by a nun named Beth Burns in Santa Ana, California. She started SJBC in the basement of her church. She raised enough money to open a dance studio in Santa Ana, Ca, in which it's now a multi-million-dollar facility called "The Wooden Floor" next to the bowers museum in Santa Ana, Ca. If you can please donate to this beautiful organization, I would really appreciate it as it is such a worthy cause and it saved me. They help inner city children like me learn to dance. Wow! I never would have imagined how my life would be so different if it weren't for Saint Joseph Ballet Company. I could have been part of a gang or married at an early age with kids. I was already a struggling immigrant. Credit goes to my dad, Juan, who found the ad in the yellow pages. They had kids audition for the Ballet school. We went and I remember all the kids in one room. We were so small, I asked myself, "How do we audition?" I was one of the lucky ones and made the cut. Thanks Dad!

Beth Burns saved my life and has been my role model as an inspiring and motivational positive teacher. I feel incredibly blessed she came into my life and gave me the gift of dance. She always had a warm and loving smile. She pushed us to be our best in dance and kind to one another. She taught with grace and played inspirational classical music. One of her favorites was "Wind Beneath My Wings" by Better

Midler. Imagine it's a Saturday morning at 10am and you hear the most beautiful classical music playing Mozart, Beethoven, Bach, Chopin. Thanks to SJBC, I was exposed to a new way of life including appreciation and respect from people outside my family; I imagined I was like an aristocrat listening to classical music at an early age.

At least I felt for that moment I belonged. I was somebody. I existed in the world through dance. You see, when you have lived in fear, cried a thousand tears, and only knew sadness, it is indescribable what a little glimpse of hope, beauty and kindness can do for your soul. It gave me a sense of peace while on earth.

There is a special sensation, a special feeling that I felt in the dance studio. As I held the ballet bar for the warmup I felt at peace, connected with myself, and completely focused. I forgot all my troubles. The teacher gave me notes and pushed me to perfect my steps and moves. I slowly started to get stronger with my body but also with my mind.

Dancing was my first home. I ate, slept, and breathed dance. Monday through Friday, I was in dance class after school for two to four hours. Saturdays and Sundays from 10am- 6 pm. I would take all the classes, study and do my homework in between classes and at home. Late at night I would even move the living furniture, turn on the T.V. and put on the classical channel where there were only the color stripes on the screen. That's how much I would practice and try to do crazy moves like I saw the Cirque du Soleil dancers do.

At one of the school's recitals, I gave a speech in front of all the sponsors. A gentleman named John Wood saw me speak and told my director Beth "That young lady is a beautiful dancer and should also have a beautiful smile." He sponsored five years of braces so I can have a beautiful smile. To this day I am incredibly grateful to him for showing kindness to a child he just met once. I wrote thank you letters through the school and because I have received kindness and love, I tend to be a giver, expressing love in everything I do and happy to help others.

SBJC would hold their annual showcase at the Irvine Barclay Theatre in Irvine, Ca. It was one of the most exciting events of the year. You waited for the line up to be posted to see which dances you would be in. We get to see the sketches of the designs for the show. You work all year to get better and grow. The show represented a celebration of doing something you love and hope.

One year was especially unique. I was introduced to Latin jazz. It was a completely different feel, choreography, and music. It was super exciting with lots of flavor. Our featured guest artist for the show was an upcoming artist named Poncho Sanchez! I remember meeting him, he wore his hat, had his fingers taped and he had conga drums. A couple of the top dancers and I did a photo shoot with him for the SBJC newsletter. Poncho Sanchez gave me his hat after the shoot. How impressive is that? I never would have imagined years later I'd be teaching with his music at my dance academy. I loved the Latin flavor, charisma, and soul of jazz.

Growing up in the performing arts was an amazing experience. The school would take us on road trips to see all kinds of performances from classical ballet to Cirque du Soleil. At the age of 13, I remember seeing the most captivating Argentine Tango dancers perform Stage Tango. It was the cast of Forever Tango performing at UCLA Royce Hall. I remember thinking I will do that one day; not knowing how or thinking how impossible it probably was.

I simply had hope and told myself anything is possible. I visualized myself on that stage.

CHAPTER 3

MY DANCE STORY TRAINING

A serendipitous win!

"*I believed in myself so much that I was ready to be poor and give up everything in order to one day have everything that would make me happy*" *It worked!*

The beginning stages of my dance journey were not so pleasant, and in fact, there are moments of confusion, unkindness, and pain. When you are a young adult, you're still discovering so much about yourself in life, and for me, I was conflicted about my passion, which is dance, and outside pressure to do the right thing and get a career. In this initial stage of my journey, I chose to do the "right thing" and I quit dancing. I went to college and decided to be a lawyer and minor in history. I'm a black and white type of person, so I'm all in or not, so when I quit dance, I completely removed myself from all dance activities and training. I was a full-time student, 18 units, six days a week. At school during the day and studying by night. I was determined to be successful at anything I did.

Growing up, I was bullied as a child. I always struggled with me image and was self-conscious. I always thought I was fat, a chubby dancer. I choose to keep to myself and focus on the task at hand, which was partially because my parents were so strict, I didn't really have a social life; partly because I couldn't go to the movies with just my school mates; my mom or my little brother Kevin had to come too. It was so embarrassing. I never got to be a kid. I remember I went to a sleep-over maybe three times at most. But now, as an adult, I appreciate that my mom was overprotective. It helped keep me whole, innocent and a special gem of a lady. Like a rare diamond. I lived in my own little box and wasn't exposed to bad influences. Even pop culture was not so present in my life. I was so focused on classical dance and the performing arts. I didn't have time for the real world and what's popular, what's trending or what's cool.

While in college, there was one instance where I went to a friend's birthday at JC Fandango nightclub in Anaheim, Ca. They had two rooms, one of them was rock en Espanol, the other had a live Salsa band. We were able to walk around both rooms and when I went to the salsa room, my girlfriends and I went onto the middle of the dance floor to dance merengue and I started twirling and just dancing. It was my first-time having fun in a long time outside of school. The band played the next song, and a young man came to ask me to dance.

Now I realize he thought I knew how to dance Salsa, but I didn't even know what that was. I said yes, and of course did all the wrong things I could have done, turned the wrong way, doing my own thing, but he noticed I was a dancer and took me outside, showed me the salsa basic and the right turn. This is my first-time knowing salsa dancing existed even though I grew up in Bolivia with tropical music and danced at my family gatherings. After doing a couple of the basics, we went back inside and there was another song, which I recognize to this day. It was "Idilio" by Willie Colon. It was simply perfect, and it was simply magical. I was dancing Salsa.

It was so much fun, and the young man asked me to practice with him. He needed a practice partner to practice Salsa moves. Of course, that was the most ridiculous thing I've ever heard, and I didn't quite understand what that meant, but I thought how much I missed dancing, and this could be a good way for me to have a little bit of dance back in my life. So, I was officially introduced to the world of Salsa and months later, during a Salsa night at the world-famous Mayan in Los Angeles, as I'm in the alley getting some air outside, a professional dancer greets me by asking me "Can you do the splits?" I looked up at him without saying anything, raised my leg up; he catches my leg, lunges, and there I am doing the splits. That was my introduction to Alex da Silva.

In 2002, a couple of months later, he asked me to compete with him at The World Mayan Salsa competition. I had no idea what I was getting myself into. I thought, "Nobody knows me. It's all good. Why not? It should be fun and over the summer it's a good activity or hobby for me to do while studying and stressed out with school projects." I wasn't aware there were different divisions such as amateur, semi-pro and professional. I had no idea that any of that existed or that I even had a choice. In the finals, I remember wearing a red dress I bought for $20. I put one line of studs across the front of my dress and wore a red rose in my hair. My first Salsa competition; the crazy thing is I had unknowingly competed as a professional because my partner was a professional and by default, I became a professional. We won first place!

That moment completely changed the course of my life.

I realize now how creative I was. Even in my first competition, I was able to create moves that I felt I could execute because of my training and talent. All those years of hard work, sacrifice, and dedication since the age of six led to that moment. I realized how much I missed dance in my life and how much I loved to dance.

As world champions, we got invited to perform and teach around the world. In the blink of an eye, I'm living a completely different life. I struggled and was so conflicted that I decided to talk to my college counselor to get some advice. She said nobody really gets this kind of unique opportunity and you should enjoy it for the summer and resume school in the fall.

Of course, we all know that never happened.

When I decided to become a professional, the best advice I received was to contact all the current top professional Salsa women in the industry at the time and tell them that I want to become a professional dancer and ask them what advice they had for me. Most of them responded, whether I met with them for coffee or via a phone call. I was so appreciative of their time and advice. It's funny because years later, I found out that one of them said, "Oh she's not going to make it." It stuns me that there are people in this world that genuinely don't want the best for somebody and genuinely don't support another human being.

But of course, there are wonderful people out there that genuinely do want your success and want to be there for you. That's the kind of person I am. One particularly important piece of advice all of the women were adamant about was to never get involved romantically with your professional dance partner. Thanks ladies. By me embracing this philosophy and staying true to it, I'm grateful I've had successful partnerships and can be friends and they completely respect me as a woman and what I've accomplished, and of course, everything we accomplished together and my appreciation for them dancing with me.

I believe that it definitely makes a big difference in one's life, when making decisions and taking risks, to have your family's love and support for you to know they are there for you no matter what, they'll be there to pick you up.

In every industry there are going to be some bad apples. One of my partners, especially in my beginning stages, I was so shocked, and of course naïve about so many things that I stayed quiet and didn't quite know what to do when I witnessed things. For example, we would be at an event and sometimes we would share the same room, two beds, and I would walk in, and he would be there with a random girl and in bed. Of course, I just pretended I was alone and went to bed. Then just the harshness of a partner putting you down and being sarcastic or, at your expense during a workshop, there is a joke about demeaning women. There was nothing anybody else can do and I had no voice. I didn't know how to express that I felt uncomfortable, so I'd stay quiet. Sometimes, it gets sad.

In the middle of all this, as I'm traveling, there is so much success and competing and winning more championships and just enjoying the fruits of my labor, a really good friend of mine passed away. That impacted my journey because I had to hide it, at least I had chosen to hide it. I didn't want anybody to know my sadness and my pain during this phase. It definitely made me stronger and helped me realize that life is too shotty and we should all pursue our dreams and do what we love and be who we want to be because you never know when it's your time.

At that moment, I gave myself permission to become the master of me. What that meant for me was to let go of negativity and ignore people that bully you and surround myself with amazing mentors, coaches, dance acquaintances, and family and friends.

In the dance world, in my beginning stages, I definitely realize I was only made fun of because I had such a strong ballet background. I used to dance with tremendous turnout in my feet. For example, so you can imagine, doing the Salsa basic with turned-out feet. That's just what my body mechanics were and so I danced like that, and I didn't realize that people would comment and initially bring me down and say, "that's not Salsa," and so on, but I had a certain vision for myself, and I stuck to it against all odds of what in that moment was considered street Salsa dancing. I was truly fortunate and I'm immensely proud of myself for being who I wanted to portray and the dancer I wanted to be. For that reason, I brought lines and more beautiful turns, stylistic ideas, and tricks to open the forum for more creativity and more techniques in our beautiful salsa and Latin dances.

It's a blessing to see others take after me and go take a ballet class and work on their connection in becoming better dancers, not just people who dance Salsa at the nightclubs, but truly be able to take our beautiful dance to the next level. I've had amazing coaches who have helped me do that through International Latin, Argentine Tango, and my classical dance background.

One of my wonderful and favorite mentors and coaches in Latin dance was Melissa Dexter. She comes from old school Latin dance training, and she was really the first person to introduce me to the artwork of Latin dance and partner-work. She helped me understand the feminine way of dancing as a woman from my body position to the feeling of how I'm connecting to my partner and all these little details with the body mechanics to be able to create shapes, isolation work and weight transfer. I really felt like I went back to being a beginner with her, which I really loved. A lot of the important aspects of Latin dancing that I hadn't focused on, I was able to focus on with her, and that became my foundation.

Through executing such detailed work and understanding exactly how it all works, it started to shape, change, transform and take my dancing to a whole another level.

I've also had other wonderful mentors such as Wendy Johnson, Ron Montez, Vivica Taft, and one of the greatest, Shirley Ballas, who stated one of my favorite phrases to me while I was extremely focused on training and was really trying to get this one move. While I was really killing myself to execute this move perfectly each time, she walks by me, looks at me, smiles and says, "Smile, it's just dancing." I will never forget that. I think it's so important to remember, yes, we can work hard, but, man, enjoy it and enjoy the journey and experience and work hard, but be kind to yourself and smile while you're at it. With Shirley, I got more refined in my talent and my artistic work. She truly just has this gift to give you the particularly important technique and artwork for partner dancing. When I worked with her, we focused on perfecting technique and technical elements to be as refined and defined as the level of world class dancers, from footwork details to body mechanics, partner, and connection.

Details are what separates being good from being great. She's one of the few coaches in the world that trains at that level of detail. I remember her being so supportive, believing in my talent, so much so that I went on to work with her son and ex-husband on some choreography work in TV and film. We just really connected, and I felt, to this day, so fortunate to be able to learn from her and other top coaches as they have been wonderful role models in my character, education in dance, and in my professionalism.

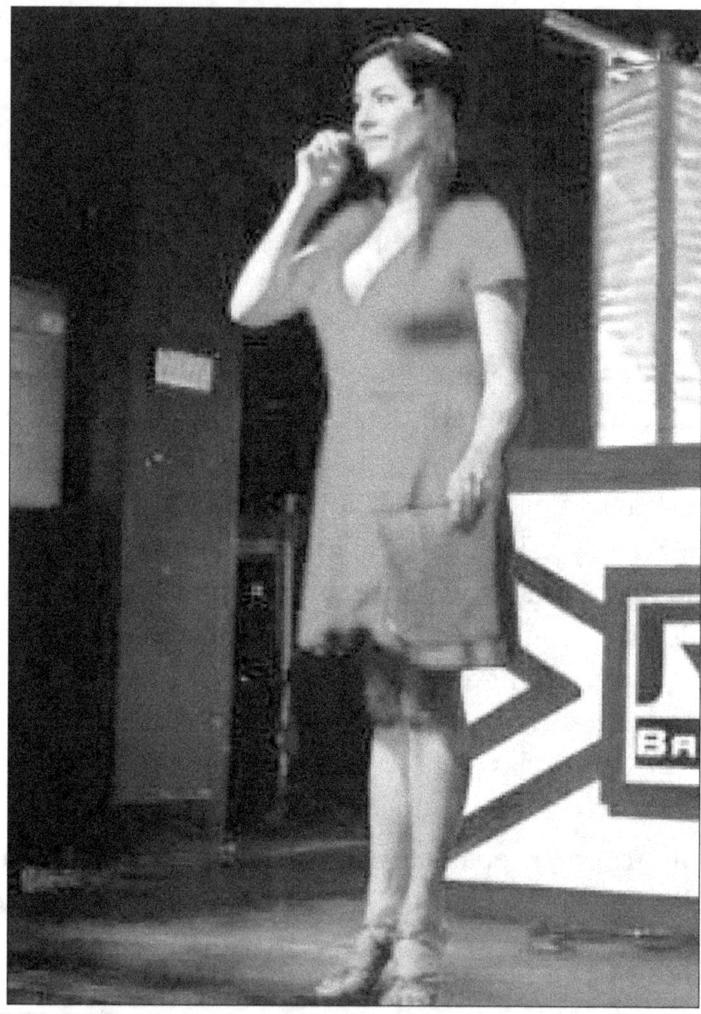

Liz Lira speaking and sharing her story, inspiring others to do what they love and treating dance as a gift that transforms lives. Local venue in Sherman Oaks.

Dance changes life brings joy and brings everlasting friendships.
~ Liz Lira

A STRONG WOMAN IS NOT JUST EQUAL, SHE'S ALSO FEMININE AND MAINTAINS A BALANCE WITH WORK, LIFE AND EXPRESSION

"Smile, It's just dancing."
~ Shirley Ballas

That's right ladies, just smile and don't worry so much. Life is like dancing. You must go with the flow.

A woman's role is to not back lead as it can negatively impact the way you connect with a partner and little things like styling that can interrupt the leaders' movements. You must be able to let go and be in your feminine energy in dancing. This is so important for women. Currently, women are dancing like men on the dance floor and potentially acting like men off the dance floor. I hate to say it, but it's true.

That's crazy. We are our own gender with wonderful complexity of masculine and feminine aspects. Don't lose your femininity. There are less and less of us left who embrace our feminine so let's share this message.

What dance brings into a woman's life outside of the dance floor is the ultimate woman: strength through femininity, confidence, passion, and happiness. I believe men want to be a gentleman, protect, and help us, and enjoy being supportive. I've seen women let their guard down on the dance floor and they just chill and embrace their role by closing their eyes and allowing the leader to guide them. There is a sense of relief and an "aha" moment that ladies start to enjoy the dance better. They reconnect with their natural intuition and can connect better with a different sex and other women.

Initially it's not that easy to stop being in control. To be vulnerable and let someone else guide you can be difficult to do if you have trust issues or are simply shy, hesitant, or afraid of your feminine side; especially women that are in powerful positions such as CEO's or other demanding "masculine" positions.

I remember a student who was a legit police officer. She walked into the studio in uniform, and I thought something bad happened. She looked at me and said she wanted to sign up for dance class. It was awesome to see her transformation. She was new to dance and excited to explore her body and sensuality through dance. We worked on Salsa and Argentine Tango. Her look started to transform. At the beginning she would wear jeans and a T-shirt, but then eventually she bought dance shoes and started to wear skirts and dresses. She started to go out dancing and was looking happier and more fulfilled. You would have never guessed she was a police officer if you saw her on the dance floor. She became a whole person, a strong woman in all aspects of her life.

There are so many positive results when a woman outside dance can simply let her guard down, focus on herself and be a little more open minded by embracing their feminine role even dressing the part, such as wearing a dress and heels. I am not saying you must but at least occasionally it's nice. Body language is everything in life. Through dance, I see substantial changes in women's physique, posture, how they walk, stand, and carry themselves with more beauty. Simple changes that do inspire a woman to act a certain way and feel more joyful, sensual, passionate, and confident.

Ladies, my question to you is: Do you want to declare who you are to the world now? How do you become a more complete person? And what do you want your role as a woman to be in dance and outside of dance? It's so important to understand your mindset and intention in all stages of life.

As for me, I've declared to embrace my femininity in all aspects. I want to have it all. Feeling like a woman, and embracing my nurturing side, being a lady, more graceful, patient and loving. We can get tested. Life happens! If I ever get tested, I try my best to find the good in every situation and be patient and understanding and keep things simple. For every issue, there is a solution. I genuinely believe that. If you feel stuck or there is no way out, well, I want to tell you there is. Never settle and never give up. Dance is improvisational and we need to do our best to read our leader's guide, even if he gets off rhythm or misses a beat. We want to make it look good and stylish when we have the opportunity. Make it fun! Ladies understand your partner's role and be clear and direct in what you need. Be on the same page together and understand each other's roles. Communication is the key to any successful relationship.

Remember ladies, the guy might be leading but everyone is looking at you. It's the man's job to build the structure to make you look good.

I love embracing my feminine role by also dressing like a woman. I love heels and beautiful dresses. I want to conquer the world in six-inch heels, and most importantly, live a fulfilled life by having balance in my workplace, in my personal life, and my hobbies.

Have a little me time. I'm so lucky my hobby is dance. By creating this balance, I'm able to be happier and less stressed. The words stress, anger, hate, rage, selfish, and evil are not in my dictionary and by simply connecting to myself and my femininity through dance, I have been able to find the right partner, friendships, and they have been organic, successful, and everlasting.

Sharing love and kindness in our dance community is especially important. Kindness and respect are the foundation of my dance academy. We are all equal and share the love for dance. Actions speak louder than words. The first step is for me to be a role model. Just like in dance, knowing my role in movement is important. Dance can change the way you move off the dance floor. You may move with more grace, more confidence, and more awareness.

I also find the need to demonstrate love and kindness in character. I know sometimes the word love can be something very particular to some people, and I completely respect that, but I definitely believe that there's many types of ways of showing love, from your husband to a friend to even just your dance family.

What does the word love mean to you?

How do you express love?

If you come from a place of love and kindness to the people around you, in my experience, people will always respond better to you, whether you're in a situation of conflict or simply in a situation where you're trying to figure something out and brainstorming.

In the dance community, we're very open-minded. It's very joyful, lots of laughs, and memorable moments. Once you get the bug, you immerse yourself increasingly in the dance scene. You're officially a Salsa-holic or Bachata Lover or you get Swing Fever or even Disco or Country Fever. (You take group classes and go out dancing every day for months on end.) You're feeling good, happier, more kind, love yourself and others. Dance can affect your life daily; from the moment you wake up, to your morning tasks and going to work, your work environment, and your peers. Imagine yourself being happier, more patient, less stressed, bringing joy into your workspace, going from your dance community into your own community and, of course, into your family life, and how you treat your loved ones and everyone around you.

Through dance, you can receive such beautiful and memorable moments that you can also experience with complete strangers all the while having so much fun and inspiring one another and allowing that to shape your life. Not judging a book by its cover is a lesson I had to work on and be patient with myself because not judging is also being able to trust. To trust, obviously, is something that should be earned and it's not easy to give people trust. But we can certainly give someone a chance.

So, through dance, as we're dancing with different dance partners, we learn to connect with different people of all different walks of life and to take that mindset in the outside world, where you first start by seeing the best in someone and not judging people, is a difficult but incredibly important thing to do. It's giving someone a chance and learning about them in a safe environment on the dance floor and then possibly off the dance floor. With the skill of learning to connect with someone, it can be applied in the workplace, social settings, supermarket, gym, etc. In partner dancing, I believe acquiring that skill makes you more open to diverse cultures, languages, and people with which you wouldn't traditionally connect.

Lastly, I want to say that you need to give yourself a chance. Once you step onto the dance floor, you just completely set yourself up to improve as a dancer, as a person, and as a human being. Most importantly, you give yourself a chance to be good and see the good in others on and off the dance floor.

CHAPTER 5

MEN'S LEADERSHIP IN DANCE

"When a body moves, it's the most revealing thing. Dance for me a minute, and I'll tell you who you are."
~ Mikhail Baryshnikov

The definition of a leader in partner dancing is a leader that must master his dance rhythms and the art of partner dancing.

The leader's role is that he is confident in himself and knows exactly how to properly guide the partner. He can improvise and have his own style without disrupting the partner, and to be able to enhance the partner's dancing and experience.

Here are four steps to ensure you are an amazing leader.

1. Know your rhythm of the dance, the counts of the basic steps. You are able to break it down by yourself without a partner. Master your steps. Counting in dance is so important because it will haunt you later in your journey, as you advance, if you can't follow and lead the counts. You'll struggle to stay on the beat and not have a good flow with your partner while social dancing. Better to practice counting from the beginning.

2. Understand how your weight and frame affects the partner in motion. You must be confident with your role first

before you can try to focus on the partner. This means you should practice on your own and look at all aspects of your movements from head to toe.

3. Be aware of your technique. You don't need to be in a competition or even perform, but it's important you know basic technique, such as foot and leg placement, alignment, posture, balance, hand mechanics in transition from one move to the other and most importantly, so you don't get injured or injure your partner.

4. Test your leading skills and combinations with a professional dance instructor to get feedback and clean up any bad habits. Take notes, video tape and ask questions about why you should make a move in a certain way. Don't just copy the move. Learn how to do the move by breaking down your part first and then with a partner.

In a group class setting we ask our leaders to please escort the lady next to the partner. As silly as that sounds it works beautifully because from the very start the leader is acting as a leader and the lady is acting like a lady and enjoys being escorted. I see those lovely smiles.

In dance, a man learns to be a leader. He learns to take charge instead of being passive. He learns to become more improvisational. He learns to connect with a woman in a safe environment with the sole purpose of matching partner led moves to the shared musical experience. And these skills don't just stop on the dance floor. I've worked with many men who were shy and passive who became strong men, kind men and connected men.

✳✳✳

Dance Tips For Gentlemen

12 Tips Every Man Should Know Before Stepping onto a Dance Floor. By Francisco Martinez.

1. Keep an eye on the ball. When considering asking a lady to dance, look at her from where you're standing. Try to make eye contact and smile as you walk up to her, extend your hand, and ask her to dance with a subtle bow of the head towards her. NOTE: Try not to extend your right hand as you might walk away with a handshake instead of a dance partner.

2. Learn to strike out like a champ. If a lady says no, simply smile and say, "okay - maybe later" and quickly ask another lady to dance. Repeat until you are on the dance floor. NOTE: Avoid any comments or gestures to make up for the awkward feeling of hearing "no."

3. Look up. A woman can feel uncomfortable with a man while he is looking at his feet. From her perspective, you are looking at her body, so make sure to look up, being careful not to stare into her eyes or at her mouth.

4. Look sharp and smell fresh! A shower, mints, deodorant, and lightly scented cologne in moderation can make up for your lack of dance savvy. Make sure keep your nose, ear and body hair trimmed and clean shaven.

5. Observe the one dance rule. Only assume one dance with a lady you have invited out to the floor. When the song is done, politely ask her if she can save you another dance, and politely escort her off the dance floor.

6. Nice guy wins. Ladies will often comment on how nice a gentleman was rather than how good of a dancer he was on the floor. Your most important dance move is your smile.

7. Gauge your partner. Start your dance time together with basic, easy, and fun moves that will allow you both to relax. Increase the complexity to her ability level. Keep dips and multiple spins to ladies who you know, only attempt them if you have been professionally trained in dips. This will naturally bring out her best dancing.

8. Dance as if no one is watching. The simple truth is people are not watching you, that are watching the lady. Remember you are the stern; she is the flower. You provide the frame for her to paint the canvas.

9. Just say "NO." Although the idea of drinking before dancing may make you feel less inhibited, try to keep alcohol consumption to a minimum. It could impair your judgement and create foul breath. Do drink Gatorade or other electrolyte replenishment drink after an active night of dancing, before going to sleep. This will help avoid waking up with a headache the following morning.

10. Keep your cool. If the idea of asking a lady to dance causes you to sweat profusely, and if you know yourself sweating a lot, make sure to have a change of shirt.

11. Know your game. Like any good quarterback studies his playbook, do not assume that your moves are up to date. All great dancers receive training and instruction to stay up on their game.

12. When free styling, instead of moving your feet, work on swaying your upper body. Avoid any jerky or big movements and intermittently clap casually. You'll look like the most confident man out there!

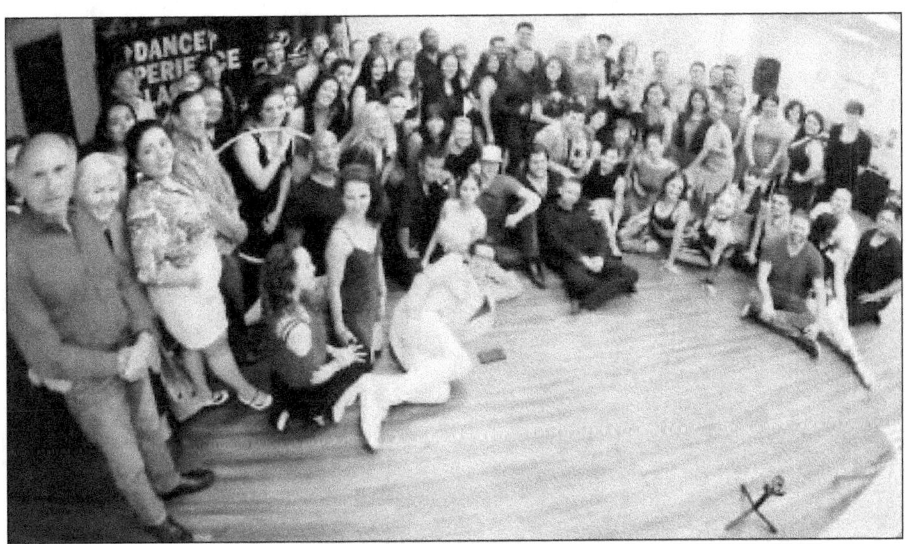

Pictures: Above Liz Lira Dance Experience First Annual in Los Angeles, Ca   A three-day event with specialty workshops from Zouk fusion to Theatre Arts (lifts and tricks). Student birthday celebrations. An exciting Salsa and Bachata Jack n Jill open level and dancing till 5AM

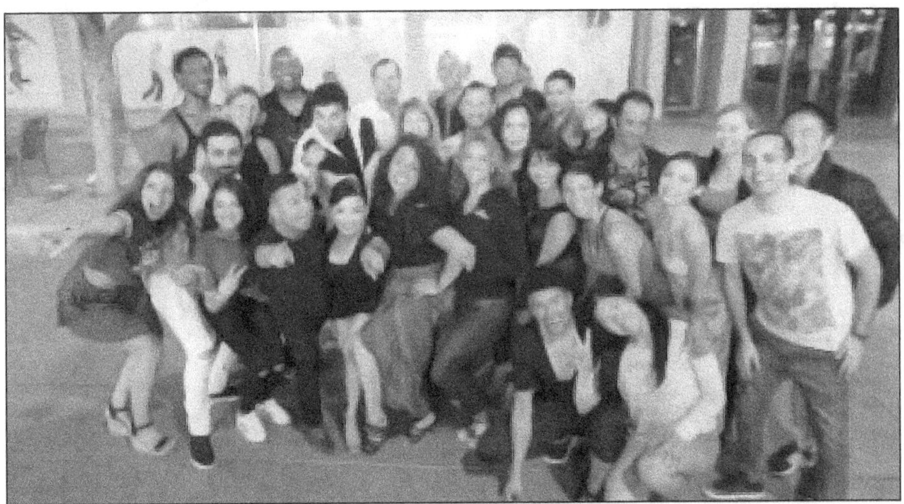

Third day birthday dinner and dancing outdoors at the famous third street promenade in Santa Monica, Ca

CHAPTER 6

CHIVALRY IN THE MODERN WORLD

"People that respect themselves will act accordingly and show their true selves in their actions towards others."
~ Liz Lira

The Art of Partner Dancing

A balanced partnership and relationship.

A gentle touch, sweet kind greeting, a shy smile, and a free soul. Simply lost in the music. It's this beautiful and unique way of communicating without saying a word with a complete stranger. There is an organic expression of the music and every movement created is one of a kind from its feeling to its form.

This is partner dancing with a new partner.

Can we connect?

In the modern age, due to the feminist movement and other things that are happening in the world, it's getting more difficult to connect to another human being, let alone meet someone new that is genuine and has good intentions. I believe that I've been able to maintain my femininity and continue to embrace my role as a woman as the years have passed, through dance. Not just putting on a dress and heels, but in embracing my nurturing, sexy, and loving self. Lately I've been paying attention to my girlfriends who are really struggling to connect with the opposite sex and vice versa. They are beautiful, successful, and super fun gals. Struggle has inspired me to draft this book and to share with them that there is this beautiful art called dance and it can help you have balance in your life and so much more.

We are slowly losing a genuine and organic way of being in our own role, masculine or feminine. Finding equality is making women become more like men and men are slowly not caring about how to be a man. Of course, there are those few wonderful gentlemen out there, but I see men who are turned off by women who are trying too hard to be like a man, and I see women turned off by passive men who don't know how to connect.

Dance has been so amazing for me to find a balance between work and my personal life. It hasn't been easy, but dance has always brought my spirits up, helped me to have a healthier lifestyle, embrace being a woman (being sensual in an elegant way) and to connect with beautiful people even if it's only for one dance.

I've worked really hard to be a strong, independent, and successful woman running my own business. At the same time, I would like to continue to connect to someone on the dance floor and off. Fortunately, I've been able to connect to the most amazing men in my life. Through dance, I've been able to continue to embrace being a woman and also share a specific way of thinking, a mindset so that I can be strong and independent, but also connect and meet genuine men or women that will be supportive and admire the way I carry on with my feminine role. For men in this day and age, in my humble opinion, I believe it's getting harder to connect to a woman, because a lot of women are becoming or acting like men (even dancing like men) and there's this power struggle that is making it exceedingly difficult for men to connect with women.

"*I want to conquer the world in six-inch heels.*"
~ Liz Lira ***

In dance class, I teach wonderful etiquette of simple ideas that are an essential part of the Liz Lira method. The first thing all students should learn is the definition of partner dancing. I always ask my students to repeat after me. Please join me in this exercise. And say out loud: Partner dancing is individual work with awareness of the partner. What does this mean exactly? On the dance floor and off the dance floor, it mean creating a perfectly balanced relationship. Yes, I come from an old-fashioned perspective. Where gentlemen open doors, court a lady, and have manners. Where ladies act properly (respect themselves in other words), understand giving power is not being less than, but being greater than because they have the choice.

Be a strong, independent, and successful woman, but don't forget your femininity and always celebrate being a woman.

A balanced relationship. Wow! What a thought.

That's what all dancers try to create on the dance floor. First, find your own balance and be in control of it. Second, give forward weight to have 60% more on the balls of your feet when you dance and 40% on the heels. Dance forward with your weight to have better balance, create connection, and because we wear heels. Afterwards, the lady simply waits for the leader for a quick second, as the leader is always going to be a second ahead of the follower, and he leans forward to suggest that we're going to start to move and as he is leading through the body, he's able to signal first before his actual first step. The lady will wait and respond as soon as there is a signal.

Roles in dance for a leader and follower:

A leader has a tough job because he needs to multitask so many variables in his role. It starts with learning his counts, steps, technique, combinations, how to lead, adjust different heights and styles of ladies, and he guides the directional changes from one move to the other and has to be musical and playfully improvise. The leader also supports the lady in a dip, and he controls the balance as ladies styling may have moves that are off balance at times. He has to be confident in himself, his repertoire, and his style. To be a great leader you have to have a healthy mindset, for example, when a lady says no, a good leader understands not to take it personally. We can take things personally and think the other person is rude when the lady genuinely needs a break, is waiting for a friend, or has to get water. A great leader knows their weaknesses and strengths and owns it. I mention this as an example because there are a lot of guys who shouldn't be doing certain moves because they could hurt their partner.

A follower is sensitive to the lead. They understand the mental approach first to give the power away because you choose to do so. I learned this the hard way. I was about to go on stage and my partner said, "If you don't follow me, I won't lift you as high as possible on the jump." This meant I wouldn't look as beautiful doing that jump trick without his support. I learned by allowing my partner to lead me he would help me look and execute the jump trick to its full potential and look beautiful. Happy to say, the jump looked great! After that, I realized I have double the power to be able to choose to be led for my own benefit. How funny is that?

The reality in our own individual mind is we want to be so strong, so independent, we don't need anyone's help and we will make it on our own. I'm definitely the last person to ask for help. Dance has been a great education in learning how to get along with diverse types of personalities, cultures, and styles. In dance, the woman learns to follow, to let go, to be in her feminine and to connect with her partner. By adding our "lost femininity" to the definition of a strong woman, we will not only succeed in the workplace but also in our relationships, our connection to our bodies, and our connection to the world around us.

A mindset for a leader and a follower is truly becoming an expert in yourself by having a clear understanding of your role. By being independently responsible for each other's role and simply being aware of each other, and allowing us to work through our own ideas, and our own strengths and weaknesses, we are able to find balance in our partnership, how we connect with one another and our energy together. This is one of the ways dance maintains a perspective of the art of chivalry, an old-fashioned relationship. It would be so awesome to bring back some of the old-fashioned etiquette between a man and a woman off the dance floor.

"*Chivalry lives in dance, throughout the world.*"
~ Liz Lira

✳✳✳

5 main points men and women should integrate from dance etiquette in dating or marriage.

1. Understand your role and strength in the relationship.

2. 60/40 finding balance by meeting in the middle without being dependent on each other.

3. The leader guides, supports, and protects the lady.

4. The follower is patient, is sensitive to their guide and doesn't anticipate when the leader is leading.

5. By owning our role and by being on the same page together, we can best sync our connection, energy, and support for one another.

> **"I love feeling my feminine self on the dance floor and off the dance floor."**
> ~ Liz Lira

✳✳✳

To some extent I believe that I do find myself to be in a more powerful position by being able to maintain my nurturing side as a woman and being able to give my partner the power to be a leader and also be supportive of his choices, all while I maintain my own ways, and my opinions are taken into consideration and respected. One word: Teamwork. In a team, everyone has a role, then the team is more likely to be successful.

I believe that dance can help a lot of single people currently. In the work place I completely support equality and if you're good at something, you should be paid what you deserve and your value.

Some people try to take that too far and that really interferes in their personal life. How does it interfere in their personal life? Well, a lot of times people forget who they are … for example, women, we give birth to children. That's such a beautiful gift and a way of showing our nurturing side and embracing our physical and just genetic being. We are not like men. I believe men sometimes are confused because they're put in a position of not really understanding where they stand and how to treat women like women, when the opposite sex is trying to be just like them or their equal. So, on paper, I think it's totally fair… if you're good at what you do, you should be respected and awarded and paid what you deserve, man or woman.

When it comes to connecting with another human being and finding love, it's important to understand our physicality and just the type of biological beings that we are. I believe dance really provides this opportunity when we go social dancing or to a dance class, and all of a sudden there's no such thing as your position in a job or you can't talk and discuss personal matters, it's simply movement and body awareness and body language, which speaks louder than words. That's something so special and it really allows a leader to learn how to lead in a partnership. A follower needs to put their guard down and be humble enough to follow. I've seen women that are CEOs and run big companies and are super strong women. When they start dancing, at the beginning, they struggle to follow because they are so used to being the leader. As they are consistent, it gets a little bit easier and, in fact, fun and they enjoy being able to be free and not carry any more responsibility than they need to. So, because of that reason, and all these obstacles that our beautiful society and the world is continuing to face, I've been inspired to start the communication and just share this message, that if you dance, you can maintain and preserve a little bit of chivalry or courtship. The art and process of simply just understanding how we can connect with another human being is an incredibly special and organic way, as I believe we are meant to connect.

Couples in dance

It's quite beautiful to see couples come to the dance class, whether it's their wedding dance or they just want to do something for fun or to connect better and so on. 99.99% of the time, when I work with a couple, the follower is the one who is always trying to guide the process. And sometimes they tell the leader what to do when they don't even have their own steps or role in order. The leader in the beginning deals with it as he is not sure what to do. As soon as the leader starts becoming more comfortable in their role and what to do, they start giving feedback themselves as well. It's hard to find the balance so both feel they are contributing while they still need to embrace their roles.

I've seen amazing results, which really come down to the same point, allowing the couple to understand their roles and give the gentleman a chance to be a leader and masculine. Allowing the woman to be feminine and sexy and be led. And by simply explaining the mindset and the approach in dance that were covered in the "5 Main Points" section of this book, men and women can integrate in their relationship or marriage. We are keeping the same counts; we have these wonderful moves that we want to do together. We have musicality and a sense of expression, there's beautiful freedom to express yourself. But to be able to do that, we need to be able to understand our roles and have a little bit of guidance and structure. By doing that, even if you're a beginner, it really changes how a couple connects with each other and how they act with each other. And sometimes, I see it can go outside of dance, and that's when it's so much more beautiful. For me, for example, I've been able to apply this because dance has always kept me feminine, wearing dresses and heels, and I love being girly. That doesn't mean if you don't like being girly you cannot be open to dancing. I can share my experience that by embracing my role of the dance floor, I've been able to find the most amazing and forever lasting friends, and most importantly, my significant other. And that's just the true blessing of finding that balance, that most men and women lack in this society, because it's just getting so confusing with differentiating roles, that there's a lot of resistance to be able to connect with another human being in this old-fashioned way in the modern world. But, in dance, you have to, to be able to lead and to follow.

Singles in dance

Case study #1 – The Macho Man

In my experience, the macho man is a person who I believe secretly wants to dance, but comes off as, "I don't want to dance. It's going to make me look ridiculous." Or he's shy and doesn't feel comfortable around people watching him. I remember an instance when I had finally convinced a student to come and try dancing, and he was extraordinarily strong about being a man, and men don't dance, and he is going to give it a shot. During the class, I can tell he was so uncomfortable. He would ask questions that were ahead of his skill level, but still was trying to, I guess, get it quickly. He would act a little bit rude towards me and some of the girls because he didn't know how to act around people, and because he didn't know what he was doing, he felt completely uncomfortable. At least he tried it.

As he went along in the class, I talked to him afterwards and he mentioned how it was particularly challenging and he's definitely out of his comfort zone and doesn't know how he feels. As he continued to train, his guard started to come down and became a little bit more open. Still, it was a difficult process to accept that it's okay for people to be around you. That at the end, everybody's worried about themselves, and really, they're not really watching you and what you're doing, unless you're dancing with them. As he began to notice that it's all about him and his experience and his individual journey, he slowly came around and became more patient, a little kinder, and started to like to dance.

Ten years later, I saw him again. He came up to me and said, "I just wanted to thank you for being so patient with me when I first started taking classes with you. I was a total jerk and rude and you were so gracious and really helped me get through it and become a better person out of it." When he said those words to me, that meant so much, because I believe through dance, we have an opportunity to show kindness to other people and to give people a chance. Having had the opportunity to travel the world and to give people a chance. Having had the opportunity to travel the world and meet so many beautiful people and cultures and ways of living and lifestyles, I realized you really can't judge a book by its cover, even though sometimes that's so hard to remember. See within you the better person you can be, as it's so easy that someone else can judge you as well so quickly without really knowing you.

So, for this macho man, he's now dancing, enjoying the social dance scene, and traveling to beautiful events and congresses. The best part is he is a better person because he chose to give dance a chance.

Case Study #2 – Newly Divorced

One of the most difficult moments in a marriage is divorce, and sadly, in this generation, it's becoming increasingly common.

I've been extremely fortunate that my parents are still together and married and have always strived to reach that goal. Nowadays it seems like a dream, but one thing I do know from my experience is that dreams come true. No matter how impossible they may seem. However, I have encountered people that come to me and say, "I just got a divorce, and want to do something different, fun and take my mind off things. I've always wanted to dance but my parents didn't let me."

When I teach a newly divorced person, I get a sense of sadness, sometimes guilt, stress and they are a little bit lost. I strongly believe that dance can prevent divorce, whether it's one-sided (that one of them dances and learns to appreciate and be patient with their significant other) or they both dance, but to have success in life, ultimately you need trust and you can learn that on the dance floor.

As sad as I get meeting a newly divorced person, for them to find dance, I believe, is such a wonderful next step to finding themselves, meeting new people, and bringing joy and laughter into their lives. A newly divorced woman I met, for example, somehow had forgotten her femininity, how to be sexy. She dressed completely conservatively, and perhaps a little bit shy, and didn't really know who she was, a part of her identity had been lost. She was so focused on her family and kids, she forgot about herself. I've seen many other divorced women share these same sentiments.

Once they find dance, and they start moving in a feminine way, meeting attractive, beautiful people inside and out, things change. They develop the freedom and creativity to rebuild an identity. Sometimes things change just because she's being introduced to heels, wearing a dress, and sharing laughter and joy! I get excited for them.

Of course, I'm sensitive to their recent experience, and perhaps they're still in the healing process. Even though I'm a teacher, I still like to connect with all students as a human being and be there for them as much as I can. I let them know that if they need any support, not only am I there, but we are all there for them, our dance family.

As they are starting class, they are exploring their movements, sensuality, elegance, and grace, and at the same time, their fire and energy. Women may have a sense of attitude or, as we say sometimes, you know, being like a diva or a princess, or a sex warrior or something feminine. It's like playing a character. So, I always tell women that I feel it's playing a character and being confident and seductive, and a beautiful salsa goddess.

I work on their mindset, and for them to understand they can initially separate who they are as a shy, conservative (that's me) person, to a different person on the dance floor. Eventually, they can integrate the two personas on or off the dance floor as one.

It might be the way they've been disciplined growing up and that's totally fine. We all can respect that, but in the arts (music, acting and dance), you are open to becoming a character, and portraying that character in its true form. Latin dancing, for a woman, is being seductive, sensual, sexy, confident, sharp, and portraying this not only through your wardrobe, but also your movement, creating a feeling, expressing yourself and that's genuinely exciting.

I see these former divorcees get their groove back!

✳✳✳

"My wife will divorce me if I don't learn to dance."
Wow! The first time I heard this I was shocked. I could not believe this could happen. It did. The older gentleman secretly

took dance classes with me for a couple of months and planned a trip to a topical Latin destination to surprise his wife and they stayed together. Bravo!

Case Study #3 Loves to dance and can't date in the dance scene but has trouble dating a non-dancer.

One of the hardest parts in the dating scene, when you love to dance, is to be single and to really love dance, but you choose not to date a dancer, that way you're not part of any drama or you know, end up seeing your ex everywhere at all these events. At the same time, you're having trouble connecting to a non-dancer. A normal person we say and this one's a tough place to be.

My experience with so many dancers out there is that sometimes they choose dance over their love life.

It's difficult to come by because I believe you should have it all and having it all takes time and a process. From a women's point of view, choosing not to date a dancer usually comes from advice from someone whose had an unpleasant experience, or it comes from someone of status like the professional women who advised me at a younger age not to date my dance partner.

Of course, I took that as not to date anybody who dances period. It was the best advice I could have received in my early stages. This is some advice I'd pass on and still continue to do so. Of course, love happens anywhere, anytime, but regardless, just like getting to know any new person in your life, you should take your time and really get to know them.

The next thing is not dating the scene is, I hear time and time throughout the years of wonderful, beautiful women who come into the scene, and they love it. They're having a great time. They're totally new, don't really know anybody, and they go out dancing and there's this one Rico Suave guy who tries to teach them and kind of dance with them and sweeps them off their feet, and they end up maybe dating or going out with them and it's such a short period that last and then these guys, which there are quite a few, unfortunately, move on to the next woman. Not all guys are bad, or have bad intentions, but in this case, men of these sorts use women to play around and have fun, taking advantage of new women and they become a victim to them. That really sucks, because as I talk to women, and get to know where they're coming from and why they stopped dancing, one of the main things I hear is "I met a guy, he broke my heart."

Or they say, I had a terrible experience with a guy in the scene, teacher, DJ, or a promoter and then they don't say anything about it. They are too embarrassed to even talk about it, or they don't know anybody that they can talk to, and that breaks my heart. I think it's unacceptable and this is one of the few reasons why it ruins new people, or dancers in the scene to be able to have/create/build a relationship, with another person because of some bad apples, or jerks in the scene.

I've mentioned there are a lot of great guys in the scene that are super-gentlemanly and awesome, but you must get to know someone, even outside of dance. You should take your time.

So, for singles in the dating scene now, and the other way around with men, dancing, initially in the very beginning it's really a challenge. And probably the men have it the most difficult in the beginning stages as they have to learn to move, become somewhat graceful, develop range of motion. Sometimes guys work out, they're super strong, muscular, but then they can't really move and lack fluidity in their body movement. And then next, they have to learn and remember counts and moves and steps and learn how to guide a lady, and there's just so many responsibilities in the very, very beginning stages for a man who's learning to dance.

And in the scene, men, I think, more or less don't really know what to do, but I have heard a lot of feedback from gentleman that they dance to meet women, and that's fair. And that's honest, and I've also met men that just want to dance because they love music. They love the arts, they love the culture, or they're born into that cultural background, or they just kind of love dancing. It feels good, it's a great work-out experience and they genuinely just want to dance.

So, there's this nice challenge that we face as we love to dance, but yet it's hard to get to know a person in the scene when there are some bad apples ruining it for the good guys. And for men, the other effect of this, that is wonderful, is the opportunity to lead 100%. And finding that confidence in the dance world where they get to be the guide and support and of course protect the women. And that's such a great thing, I think experience, because the way society is now, men are so muted to actually be men, because they don't want to suddenly have a sexual harassment lawsuit against them. Or, you know, a woman said they did something to them, and it just can become so out of control. Sometimes these things happen and are tragic but there's also cases of false accusation and some men seem scared to act with anything in their life.

But I do see there's lots of hope through dance, because first of all, you're not necessarily having a conversation with the person. So, I think men feel if they at least know how to decently lead, and they have a repertoire, and can follow the music with musicality and counts and timing, then they can build confidence. And when they have the experience of dancing with women, and the women have an enjoyable time, men often express joy and confidence.

✶✶✶

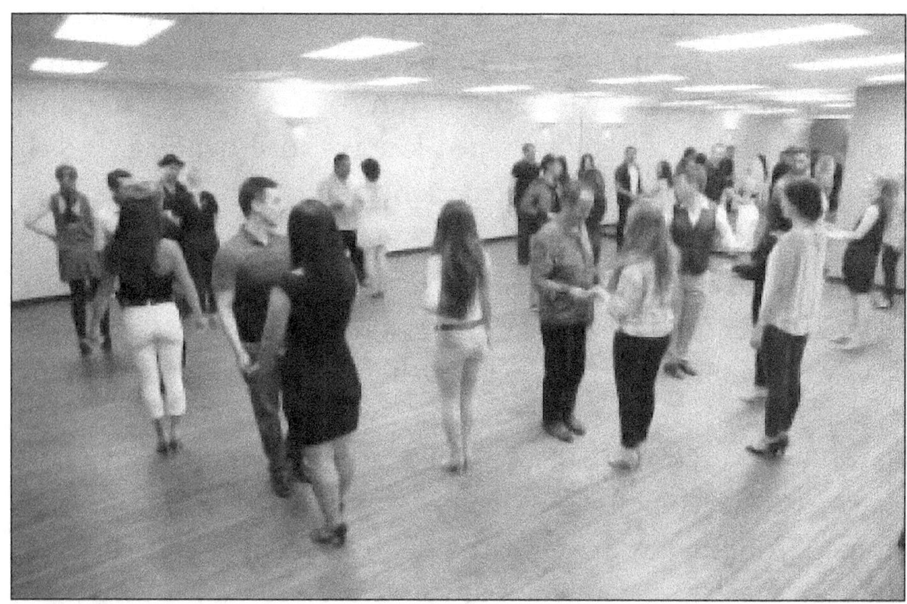

Liz Lira Dance Academy Group Classes in West Los Angeles, CA

CHAPTER 7

DANCE BENEFITS & OUTCOMES

Dance does so many good things for your brain and body.

Partner dancing does so many good things for your relationships, trust, and connection.

Latin partner dancing does better things for your brain, your body, and your soul. Because the music moves you like no other.

So, here's some things you should know about how dance makes you a better person. This is the scientific part of my book. Ready? Here we go.

Dance gives you an instant positive mood

A 2014 study in the *European Journal of Sport Science* showed that recreational dancers showed positive mood changes when they started dancing which continued after the dance. Some research studies show elevations in the feel-good neurotransmitter serotonin, while others show elevations in the rewarding neurotransmitter dopamine. Either way, it's good for you and you want to keep doing it because it feels good!

Dance and the brain

Dance requires complex mental coordination. An article published in *Scientific American* by a Columbia University Neuroscientist revealed "synchronizing music and movement-dance essentially – constitutes a "pleasure double play" as music stimulates the brain's reward centers, while dance activates the sensory and motor circuits. So, when you dance, your body and YOUR BRAIN are getting a workout!!

Research scientists have used brain imaging to identify regions in the brain that contribute to dance performance and dance learning. Per an article from Harvard Medical School, Department of Neurobiology, the brain regions involved in dance include the motor cortex, the somatosensory cortex, the basal ganglia, and the cerebellum. These brain areas assist with control, planning and execution of voluntary movement, hand-eye coordination, coordination of smooth movement and organizing complex motor actions.

Other scientists have studied what dance does TO your brain. A 2003 study in the *New England Journal of Medicine* stated that dance can decidedly improve brain health. It can help with dementia in the elderly by increasing mental effort and engaging in social interaction. Other studies show dance, for anyone, can improve mood, improve visual recognition and decision making, reduce stress, increase the feel-good hormone and neurotransmitter serotonin, and can help with spatial recognition and memory.

Dancing reduces anxiety and depression

The expressive power of movement, also known as dance, can reduce anxiety.

Dance can be a way to cope with the daily stressors or traumas; a form of stress management that can be employed anytime. Dance psychologists note that dance therapy is a way to decrease tension held in the body and overcome isolation, both occurring because of past traumas and bad experiences.

Researchers Leste and Rust (1990, 1984) did a study where they assigned patients who had anxiety to be in one of four; an exercise class, a music class, a math class, and a dance class. Of the four, only the dance class significantly reduced anxiety.

Dance is a form of exercise that involves movement with self-expression.

It's more than just exercise. It's art and connection meets exercise.

✳✳✳

Dance helps improve your physical body "Dance furthers the physical and emotional integration of the individual." ~ Bunny

Dance provides great benefits to the body. It helps with weight loss, it's a quick burst cardio workout, speeds up metabolism, improves body posture, strength, and conditioning, enhances bone strength, flexibility, breathing, coordination, and other attributes. And dancing makes the person really think about what they're doing, allowing new connections between the neurons while you learn steps, technique, and combinations (brain and body).

Testimonial

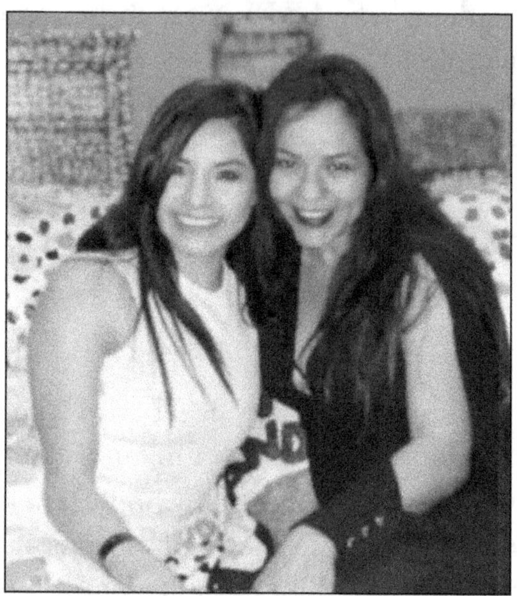

Liz Lira and Mahiely Woodbine at LA Fashion Week, Los Angeles, Ca

When I saw Liz Lira dance at the Monsoon competition in Santa Monica, Ca I was too scared to tell her I was there. I couldn't believe what I witnessed. Her every calculated move made her dance partner look sensational. Her quick but sexy slow down at the end of her every turn drew the crowd into a louder and louder roar of awe. Her long slender arms, caressing her partner's face and slowly feeling her body made you feel alive. Her elegant pointy feet barely touching the floor and gliding across the room filled the place with prestige. The glimpse of her beautiful warm smile swiftly brushed by her semi-wet sexy black hair made me incapable of blinking. Her dancing builds such enormous anticipation and the best part about Liz Lira is …. Her grand finale!!!! She never disappoints!!! Her specialty spin and her acrobatic moves in the air are better than seeing fireworks on the 4th of July! She is the firework!! Always ending with a BLAST. The rest is HISTORE!!! All praise to this sensation named Liz Lira "The Queen of Salsa Dance!!!" UNA LATINA!!!! Show the world what we are Liz!!

- Mahiely Garcia

CHAPTER 8

THE LIZ LIRA METHOD

The Art of Partner Dancing

Be present and give body weight to partner 60/40 but don't be dependent on the partner ~ Liz Lira

What did you learn from all of your experiences? How do you help people now with this method, around the world? How was this method developed? What are your plans for the future with this method and with what do you want to do?

The Liz Lira Method

Dance technique essentials are extremely important to prevent injuries, ensure awareness towards your partner, and most importantly so you can dance forever. Dancing forever is an important theme to me. Being aware of your technique and understanding the "WHY" of how to do the moves and the art of partner dancing.

I started classical dance when I was six, trained six to seven days a week for a good 15 years. As a youth/ adult I transitioned into Salsa, International Latin, and Argentine Tango at a professional level. Continued another 23 years plus with intense coaching, training everyday inside the dance studio. Let's not forget the numerous championships I've participated in.

Committing myself fully to all these amazing dance genres and living, eating, breathing, sleeping all these styles and every day training at the dance studio and understanding every single aspect that differentiate these styles, their characterizations, their story, their origin, and every single aspect that brings them together or what they share in common.

The Liz Lira method is my full commitment and devotion to dance as a professional dancer, choreographer, and artist. My main purpose of The Liz Lira method is to figure out how we can dance forever. That meant that I have to be completely aware of what I'm doing, how I'm doing it. Not only understanding the women's role, as a follower, but also understanding the work and technicalities of my partner, the leader. How he is supposed to support me so that I can understand what I need and what my partner needs. Most importantly, to be safe in my training individually and with a partner by breaking things down to the smallest detail.

For example, a simple thing like understanding weight distribution and the embrace from dance styles such as salsa and Argentine tango are day and night (completely different) in embrace, weight placement of the couple and lead and follow techniques. If you utterly understand how this works and find the patience to do the work in slow motion and really break it down, slowly becoming the master of you. It is so important at any level from just wanting to be a good social dancer to professional. I believe learning the foundation of a dance is extremely important. Learning Liz Lira foundation means writing down the counts of every move, terminology of footwork or moves, styling options for leader and follower after mastering the basics with music, body rhythm (hips figure eight, shoulder rolls, rib cage and body isolations) and musicality. By being able to master the work and physically doing the dances, whether it's competing both social aspect of them, practicing and getting coaching, it's super important.

Especially so that you don't develop bad habits or injure yourself or your partner.

I created this method so that I can impact more dancers to be safe, efficient and be a confident dancer. Knowledge is everything in anything we do in life. So, I'm combining my thirty plus years of experience, knowledge, education, teaching around the globe performing these beautiful styles.

Here in the USA and internationally it's really been important to me to pass my knowledge and the Liz Lira method understanding your body mechanisms of a high-level technique for each distinctive style of dance. I really want to emphasize the word "understanding."

"Sometimes social dancers just get the quick fix, and they copy the moves but don't learn how to do the moves."

I received tremendous feedback for my teaching skills because of this because I can take a non-dancer and know exactly what they'll need, the tools that they'll need. I can take a ballerina and she may want to learn Tango. I'll know exactly how to guide her and how to differentiate ballet with Argentine Tango, but yet along how to use some of the skills she already has. Have dancers that want to compete in Salsa or Latin dance, since I've done it with all confidence, I can show them the way. Create a training platform, schedule with goals and deadlines so that way we can achieve the goal and most importantly, their dreams.

So, this method has been developing throughout so many years as I've been able to spend numerous hours in training and coaching, learning, studying, and dancing physically. Doing that heave work of training.

My plans for the future for this wonderful Liz Lira Method is to share it online via my online course and just share as much as I can in all aspects. Whether it's from beginners to current dancers, social dancers, competitors, performers, or even teachers that would like to teach my approach because there's also a mindset of positivity and that's the way I've been able to learn. I, of course, love being pushed and challenged, but not to the extent where somebody's putting me down, bringing me down, or making me feel bad about myself, about my body or talent. Rather I have always responded better with positivity, encouragement, having goals and being motivated and of course, having role models that I can look up to and be inspired by.

The Liz Lira Method Off the Dance Floor

"We should have it all! Balance is key to a stress-free life"
~ Liz Lira

The power of dance is that it will transform all aspects of your life. Some examples include your lifestyle (wearing new clothes that reflect your personality for example), self-esteem is another example (feeling more confident as you continue to dance and naturally becomes a part of you), or even the way you exercise (such as ditching the gym because dancing is so much fun). You burn calories while you are having a fun time. Recovering from illness or tragic occurrence in your life. I personally have had a close friend pass away and dancing kept me going. Your inner self, if you bring yourself down, perhaps you tend to be negative. In dance everyone is happy and smiles. The music is vibrant, and the teachers are lots of fun and positive.

Many people say that your past will shape who you are now and who you are going to be in the future. Many people say that your past will make you who you are now, perhaps even in the future. The question I want to ask you is: Who do you want to be as a person?

Yes, we agree life is short. Time flies. That's something that I've worked hard to master. To be the expert in me. I want to give you this gift to understand and realize that you are the master of you, and you should take control of all aspects of your life. Because you can!

In my journey, I've always wanted to find balance, have it all and having it all doesn't mean being rich or fancy things or materialistic stuff. Having it all, for me, is about having good health, peace of mind, no stress, no conflict with other human beings in the world. Most importantly and number one priority is being kind and loving yourself.

So, who do you want to be?

Write it down:

When you're in a group class setting or on the social dance floor, how do you have a good relationship with various people? There are sometimes language barriers, cultural differences, even the fact that you've perhaps never met someone from a different country. Dance provides this beautiful gift for people that are able to connect from different levels of society, that perhaps you would never otherwise meet if not for dancing.

In my life, I've been so fortunate and so blessed to meet the most incredible human beings in my life that have really transformed and shaped me as a person and who I want to be. Oh, that's right, who does Liz want to be? I will always come from a place of love and kindness in everything that I do. That is the root I choose for my life. What is the root you choose?

By loving myself, I'm able to share love with others. I make the choices in any decisions that I make, and I always ask myself, "Do I need this?" I look at any situation, person, or item and I think to myself, "Do I need this?" and if I don't, then I don't need it in my life, and I let it go. For example, if a person is being negative, I don't need it. So, I let that person go. I'll always be courteous and kind. But I just don't need negative energy in my life.

Some kind of technical gadget, it's super cool, it's the newest trend, highly prized. Sure it would be fun to have, but do I need it? Probably not, so I let it go. Where this has helped me, a lot is in my nutrition. Choosing good healthy foods for my well-being and to have a strong body.

As a dancer it's so tempting to just want to eat everything, because you dance all day and you're burning lots of calories. But, even then, when I'm at a restaurant, or at a market, I always look at food and read the back of the contents. First thing I ask myself is "Do I need this?" If it's a no, then I let it go.

Specifically, if it has high sodium, high sugar, high calories, I let it go. It's the simple approach of thinking. Keep it simple. Same thing in dance, the simpler and more structured you dance, the smoother and cleaner the dance is.

In a group class setting, you can ask yourself how you can have a good relationship with different types of people, which is asking yourself how you're going to act and be learning with someone new. Sometimes people don't realize the way that they are acting or coming across. Even though sometimes they mean well, maybe they don't. I'm not sure. Regardless, when you are learning something with someone, a complete stranger or your significant other, it's important to be aware, or at least be on the same page with each other's roles. As a person and mentor, it profoundly affects me when I see someone putting someone else down. I do my best through teaching to guide all students individually or with a partner to be more aware of their words and actions, by taking them to a secluded area and giving them my feedback away from the eyes of others.

For example, I had one student who constantly tells me he's a slow learner and that I needed to be really patient. He was always the slowest person in class, and it was very frustrating. He constantly continued to put himself down and gets stuck in that mindset and, of course, I'm going to have a sitdown talk with him and just tell him my perspective and recommendation.

Slowly (after speaking with him) he understood and started changing the way he thinks about himself through his approach to himself and his dancing. I spoke to him about his learning journey, because I told him that, in my experience, he's doing just fine learning at a common pace, and he simply needs to change his outlook about himself and basically stop putting himself down, start bringing himself up, and when I give him positive feedback, he should embrace it and simply understand that I'm telling him the truth, not question it, not doubt it, and certainly not doubt himself.

Along with that, both the leader and follower need to learn how to communicate in the learning journey. Just like in life, understanding where you are in life. Are you and your partner on the same page? Mistakes will happen at any level in dance training, beginner to professionals. That's the way you're going to learn, grow and become better. I've definitely learned that you'll never be perfect, so we can only strive to be the best version of yourself.

In our mindset, and the way we approach communicating a mistake or something went wrong, I highly suggest using the word "WE." For example, a partner dancing in real life makes a mistake, you simply communicate to the teacher and say "We made a mistake here. Can you help us?" In a relationship take that same approach and say how can we improve here? Every time I use this method with my dance partners or students, it's been an enormous success, even though, perhaps, it was their fault. And sometimes it was my fault, but it doesn't really matter, as long as we help each other find the best solutions and continue growing and getting better with the element that we're working on.

Time to dance and leave attitude out the door!

You come onto the dance floor with a negative mindset, or perhaps you've had a stressful day, you'll be disconnected for a while. Just for the sake of your experience and your partner's experience, come in with a positive mindset. A lot of times students say, "This is my happy place. I feel like I can put my guard down. It's like a family here." That's such a beautiful gift. So, continue to embrace going into dancing with positivity, with a good attitude and with humility.

Confidence to me is something that we can always strive to have. To be as confident as we can in any scenario in dance or outside of dance. Dance provides confidence to simply love yourself, love your body, and embrace your journey while you have fun. That's the beauty of the experience of dancing, being free and expressing yourself and the main key here, like anything in life, is confidence will happen when you are knowledgeable about what you're doing and humble.

There's a lot of people that are showoffs. For example, in the middle of the social dance floor, they will stop dancing with their partner to try to teach them or correct them, while the music is playing, and people are dancing around them. Don't do that. I've seen it repeatedly, and it's not appropriate. If you're on the dance floor, simply continue dancing. Make the best of it. Enjoy the experience and your partner, but don't stop and start teaching or correcting your partner. Confidence outside of dance is remarkably interesting because when you start dancing, you're so new to that movement, and frightened to approach people. You think people are constantly watching you and it could be a little bit nerve wracking. Surely, but slowly, you build your confidence in dance and what you're doing as a leader or follower, the more you dance. The countless times I have seen my students become more confident outside of the studio and they even tell me, such as simple things from better posture or their approach to doing tasks or in the workplace, and it shows that their attitude is more positive. They are more relaxed and happier.

Through dance you can have a healthier lifestyle; burn calories, lose weight, reduce stress, learn to be more coordinated, be more social, embrace yourself. It can easily transform your life as a whole and as you keep learning and getting better, you will discover so much more about yourself and about life. You're able to take that outside of the dance studio into your life and just become better, implementing some ways from the training, perspective or even the approach of it. As a teacher, myself, I'll tell you to be kind to others, to love yourself, to be patient with yourself, and to enjoy the experience.

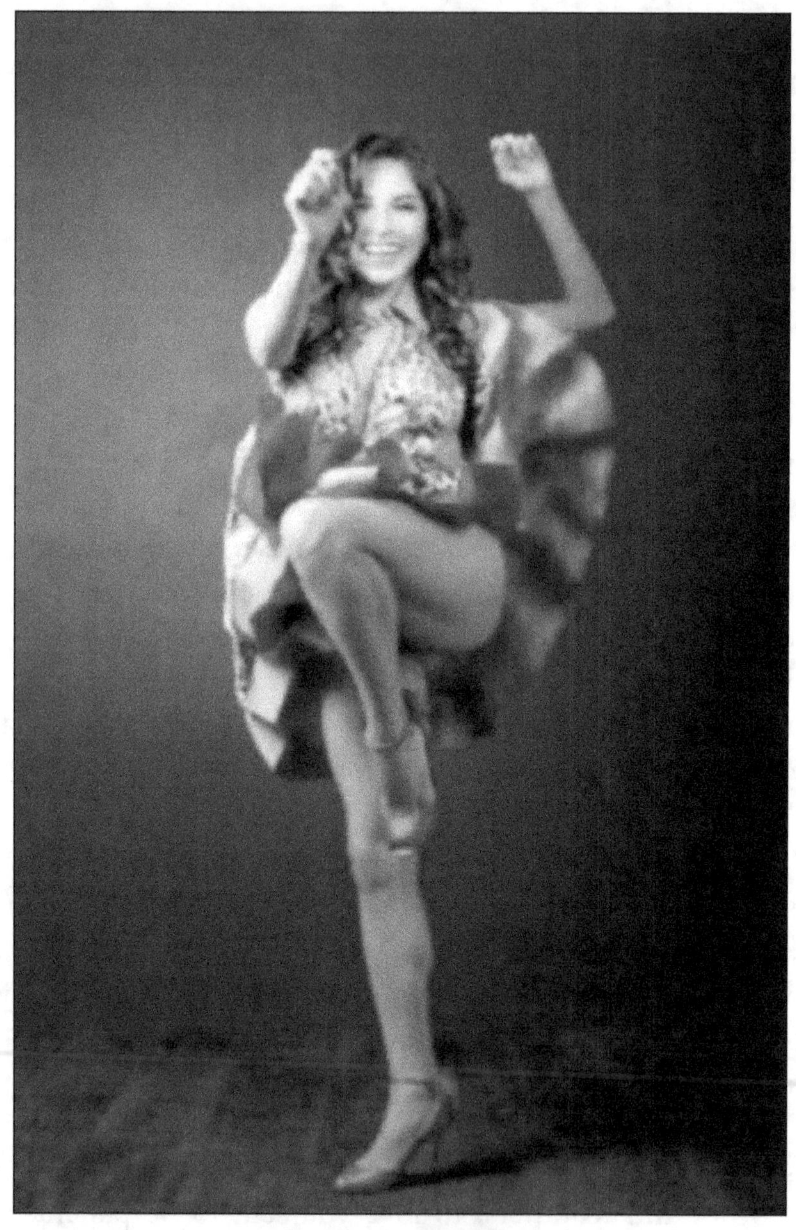

Liz Lira action shot.
Photo credit: Nishelle Walker

Dance Forever!!

Congratulations on getting to the end. It's my first time drafting a book. Just like dance found me, this book found me, and I embraced it. You can never fight your destiny, so embrace it. No matter how difficult it may seem. If you are fortunate enough to see what you are meant to be, I beg you, go for it and don't look back. You will be more successful and live a more fulfilled life, I promise. I always keep my promises.

Happy that I had the courage to challenge myself and see this book through. I look forward to enhancing and adding more content so stay tuned.

I have homework for you!

First, put on your shoes and dance. Plan your next dance class or event.

Second, embrace your destiny and don't look back.

Third, check in with your well-being and health. Your health and a happy soul makes a difference on how to carry along in your daily life. Get support or help if you feel lost.

Fourth, do not stress. It is a choice. Be the master of you! Choose not to stress. Understand that everything that needs to get done, will get done.

Fifth, say yes to doing the things you always wanted to do that you had put on hold, it's never the right time or nervous it might not work. It's your life and you are living it. So, might as well live it the way that you want.

Join my newsletter at www.lizlira.com and get a group class credit and Liz Lira Dance Academy! Email us to redeem credit. Look forward to dancing with you and welcoming you into our amazing LLDA dance family!

✳✳✳

Will you leave a book review?

Did you enjoy this book and find it useful? I would be incredibly grateful if you would post a short review and your success story on Amazon right now!

Your support makes a difference and I read and respond to all the reviews personally to make sure the next version of this book will be even better!

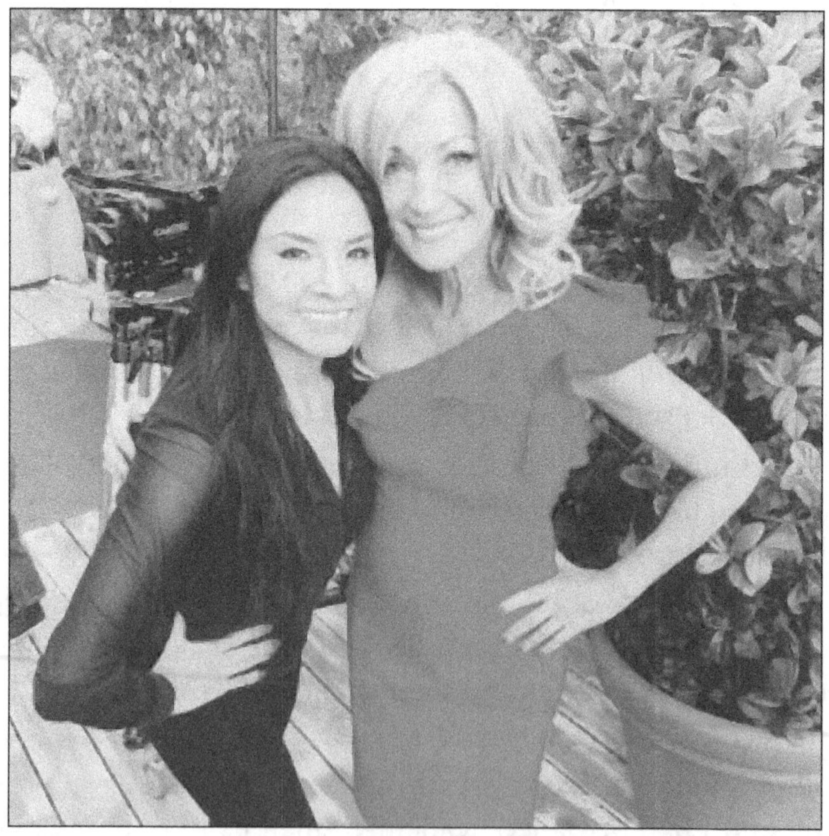

Liz Lira and Jane Seymour on the set of Friendsgiving motion picture 2019
Liz Lira – Choreographer.

LIZ LIRA SHORT BIO:

Twenty-five times world Salsa Latin Champion

2015 Grand Prix International Latin Champion

ESPN World Salsa Championship – Adjudicator

World Latin dance cup Championship – Adjudicator

So You Think You Can Dance choreographer

Dancing With The Stars choreographer

Founder and Director of Liz Lira Dance Academy

Latin Grammy's featured artist

Founder of the Liz Lira Global Foundation

Founder of Liz Lira Dance Shoes

Featured Artist and Head Judge for Feature Film, TV, and World-Wide Conferences

IMAGE AWARD of "Recognition for on-going commitment to International and local youth"

BONUS:
LIZ LIRA'S A NEW YOU THROUGH DANCE

Liz Lira's favorite breakfast, lunch, and dinner:

BREAKFAST

Banana Pancakes

- 2 eggs
- 1 Banana

Mix them together and put in the pan and walla! The healthiest pancakes ever!

LUNCH

- Quinoa
- Protein: Chicken or Fish
- Corn or cucumbers

*cook quinoa with chicken or vegetable broth

DINNER

- Ground beef
- Quinoa or rice - Grilled onions

*cook ground beef with your favorite seasonings. Cook quinoa with chicken or vegetable broth.

SNACKS

- Sprouted cashews
- JJ Virgin's All-in-one bar (chocolate mint)
- Popcorn

GENERAL DANCE TIPS FOR ALL LEVELS

The first question you should ask yourself is what are your goals?

These are some of the most popular goals:
- Be a good social dancer.
- I want to perform.
- I want to compete.
- I want to teach dance.
- Clean up my turns.
- Clean up bad habits.
- Work on my technique
- Dance with my significant other - Feel more confident.
- Build my dance repertoire.

Quick advice on your dance journey based on the years you've been dancing. My approach is safety first so we can dance forever.

Never danced before

Schedule a private lesson with a reputable instructor near you. Please learn the basic steps, counts, and start moving. Less watching, more dancing. Practice makes perfect. As soon as you can get out and social dance, I highly recommend it, as you will learn by trial and error. At this stage you get the idea of how everything works. Lots to coordinate with your role and dancing with a partner.

Danced for one to two years

Keep brushing up on your basics and technique. This is the period you can focus on building a solid foundation as a dancer and prevent yourself from developing bad habits. Focus on mastering your role according to your goals. If you really want to have consistency join a 6–12-week progressive team or a performance team.

Danced more than three years

You have experienced dancing now. It's time to check if you are becoming an overall dancer. Confident with your role as a leader or a follower. You understand the 101 rules of thumb in the world of Latin dance, and you understand the art of partner dancing. You are incorporating styling and musicality in to your dance. You are aware of your partner and what they need from you. Most importantly, you condition your body.

If you want to improve you have to put in the work, take group classes, or private lessons. Be available to practice on your own and find a practice partner.

If you have any questions or need help to customize your dance journey, reach out anytime online or via phone. I will create your own "A New You" plan.

On a side note: My wish for you

My thoughts about life.

Life is hard, life is extremely hard. I choose not to give up. I choose to be a good person. We all go through hardships, death, lies, pain, and sadness. To want to die is very extreme. Something that is very deep to me is the idea of dying. I look forward to it. I am just trying to do my best while on this earth. At a younger age, I remember how sensitive I was to the world. Perhaps you might relate, or you might know. At a noticeably youthful age when I would see somebody suffering, see someone in pain, I would cry on my own. Feel their pain. I wish the world weren't that way. I wish that people were better. How can someone get to that place of sadness or pain? The world just seems so cruel. For many years I thought, why do I deserve the things I have and would always try to bring myself down to be humble about the fact that others have less. I've always struggled with that. To this day I am extremely sensitive to people's feelings.

Change begins with us, at this very moment. Choose to be good to yourself and to others, things and to the world.

My wish and my hope for myself is to live a full life, joyful, stress free, and with lots of love. I want to inspire others to do the same. To influence people to see the good in others and to give someone a chance. To not judge a book by its cover. By starting with ourselves, we can make a change in others' lives, for the good of humanity.

This is coming from the heart. Simple sharing my thoughts. I know I am not perfect. No one is. I choose to be the best version of myself that I can be.

My wish to you is quite simple: to wake up in the morning, look at yourself in the mirror, and ask yourself, are you happy with who you are as a person? Happy in the place you live? Happy with the job you have? Happy with the relationships you have in your life and happy with your future ahead. My final wish is that you love yourself and have an open heart to love others.

Much love,

Liz Lira

www.lizlira.com – 818 929 5472

ABOUT THE AUTHOR

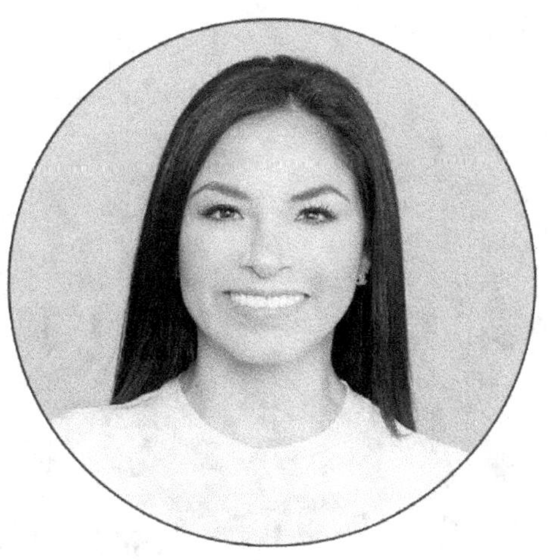

Liz Lira holds multiple World, European, and National championships as a Latin dancer. Liz is a well-known choreographer (dancing with the stars, so you think you can dance) and femininity coach, who is on a mission to help women and men connect, optimize their body, and deepen their relationships through the power of dance. As an inspirational leader, she instills confidence, and transforms lives on and off the dance floor. Her motto "Live. Love. Dance"

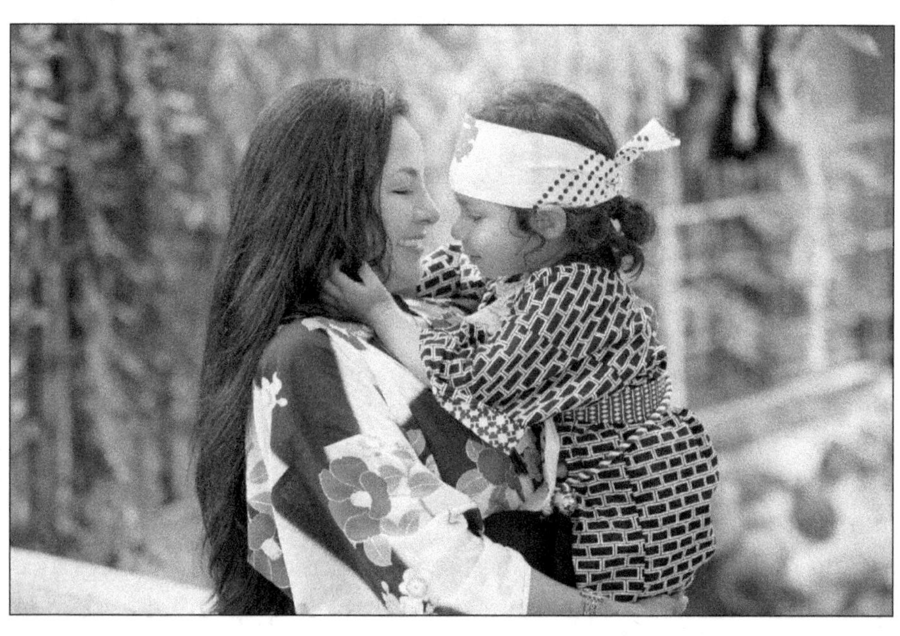